ALSO BY EVELINA WEIDMAN STERLING AND ANGIE BEST-BOSS
Living with P.C.O.S.: Polycystic Ovary Syndrome

AND BY EVELINA WEIDMAN STERLING
Having Your Baby Through Egg Donation

Budgeting *for* Infertility:

How to Bring Home a Baby
Without Breaking the Bank

EVELINA WEIDMAN STERLING &
ANGIE BEST-BOSS

A Fireside Book
Published by Simon & Schuster
New York London Toronto Sydney

This publication contains the opinions and ideas of its authors. It is intended to provide helpful and informative material on the subjects addressed in the publication. It is sold with the understanding that the authors and publisher are not engaged in rendering medical, health, legal, financial, insurance, or any other kind of personal professional services in the book. The reader should consult his or her medical, health, legal, financial, insurance, or other competent professional before adopting any of the suggestions in this book or drawing inferences from it.

No warranty is made with respect to the accuracy or completeness of the information contained herein, and the authors and publisher specifically disclaim all responsibility for any liability, loss or risk, personal or otherwise, which is incurred as a consequence, directly or indirectly, of the use and application of any of the contents of this book.

Fireside
A Division of Simon & Schuster, Inc.
1230 Avenue of the Americas
New York, NY 10020

Copyright © 2009 by Evelina Weidman Sterling and Angela Best-Boss

First Fireside trade paperback edition March 2009

FIRESIDE and colophon are registered trademarks of Simon & Schuster, Inc.

For information about special discounts for bulk purchases, please contact Simon & Schuster Special Sales at 1-800-456-6798 or business@simonandschuster.com.

Designed by Mary Austin Speaker

Manufactured in the United States of America

10 9 8 7 6 5 4 3 2 1

Library of Congress Cataloging-in-Publication Data is available

ISBN-13: 978-1-4165-6658-8
ISBN-10:   1-4165-6658-9

Contents

For my very wonderful and loving family: Dan, Ben, and Ellie.
EWS
This book is dedicated to my miracles, Kaylyn, Clara, and Katy,
who continue to fill me with wonder, joy and laughter.
AB

Acknowledgments

⁓

We gratefully acknowledge all the men and women who have faced the numerous, and sometimes seemingly insurmountable, financial barriers during their journey to bring home a baby. We appreciate your stories, advice, strength, and the motivation you gave us for writing this book. Jenna and Mike Nadeau were especially extraordinary in their willingness to share with us their personal experiences in hopes of helping others, and we congratulate them on the new addition to their family, a daughter. A big thanks goes to exceptional patient advocates Renee Whitley and Lee Rubin Collins for ensuring that we spoke with compassion and respect at all times.

We also appreciate the invaluable assistance of several highly accomplished fertility specialists who took time out of their busy schedules to help us. Dr. Sam Thatcher has been a longtime mentor, and we could not have done this without his expert advice, keen sense for perfection, and unwavering dedication to patient support and advocacy. Other fertility professionals, including Dr. James Donahue, Dr. Mark Perloe, Dr. Aniruddha Malpani, Dr. Mark P. Trolice, Dr. Janet Jaffe, and William York, RPH, gave us valuable insight on the technological aspects of treating infertility.

Because infertility is much more than a medical diagnosis, we would like to thank all the people from various professions and disciplines who truly helped us make this a comprehensive book that could speak to all regardless of their personal situation, including Mindy Berkson; Magdalena

Cogbill; Christina Gangwer; Rebekah Gholdson, Susannah Hebert; Anna Hosford, RN; Sheri and Tain Kell, Emily Klinedinst; Marcia Inhorn, PhD; Patricia Irwin Johnston; Katherine Manos, MA; Vardit Ravitsky, PhD; Wendy Simonds, PhD; Toni Siragusa; Rebeccah Devault, MBA, CPA; and Josef Woodman.

Attorneys Michael Donaldson, Liz Falker, Rhonda Orin, Sara Clay, Ruth Claiborne, Amy Wallas, and Mark McDermott were gracious in sharing their expertise as well.

We commend everyone who is working hard to provide truthful and research-based information to consumers so that they can make informed decisions. Infertility is already an incredibly stressful experience. We need to always consider the best interests of the patients above all else.

A special thank-you to our agent, Susanna Einstein, for believing in us from the beginning, and to Michelle Howry, the best editor we could hope for. We are fortunate to be a part of such a stellar team.

Finally, we would like to give a heartfelt thanks to our families—Dan, Ben, Ellie, DuWain, Kaylyn, Clara, and Katy for loving us unconditionally and supporting us throughout this process. We can't thank you enough!

Foreword

by Dr. Sam Thatcher

Infertility is not a period; it's only a comma. Most people with infertility can be successful. For women under age forty willing and able to utilize all their reproductive options, pregnancy rates approach 90 percent. For some, the path may be long, grueling, and expensive, while for others intervention may be as simple as lifestyle change. Too often it is not our lack of knowledge and technology, but access to that capability that forms the greatest barrier to fertility. Tragically, money stands between too many couples and their dream of a baby. As an analogy, what good is a drug that cured cancer if those with cancer couldn't afford it?

We all hear the great clamor about the cost of health care. No doubt it's expensive—and biased, even discriminatory. Most of the patients I see are middle-class Americans, well dressed, with two jobs, two cars, a mortgaged house, a yearly vacation, and an expensive health care insurance policy. They may have "good" insurance, but their coverage does not allow them to enter the door of a fertility clinic. Infertility therapy is considered by many insurance carriers to be *elective* and placed in the same category as cosmetic surgery or contact lenses. There's nothing about infertility that is elective, nor should there be anything elective about its therapy.

Infertility is just as crippling as other recognized diseases. The United States is in the minority of "first world" countries that mandate comprehensive fertility therapy. In our private enterprise system, insurance companies state they provide the coverage desired by the employer; therefore, it's the employer's fault. Employers in turn argue that the third-party payers have made infertility coverage unaffordable. It matters less about blame than the simple fact that the added cost for coverage of all family-building activities amounts to only pennies a day per policyholder.

Avoiding the medical cost for care of high-order multiple pregnancies resulting from overly aggressive therapy, a universally covered expense, would more than pay for the entire cost of infertility therapy, including in vitro fertilization. Patients without infertility coverage taking undue risks or inefficient treatment pathways due to incomplete coverage significantly and unnecessarily increase the overall cost of care.

Truly there is a monetary issue in insurance coverage, but to offer this as a complete explanation, or excuse, is overly simplistic. First, there exist two worlds: the fertile and the infertile. The emotional pain, isolation, and self-doubt accompanying infertility are not openly obvious and the suffering not understood by those not affected. This societal apathy leads to bias and underappreciation of the burden of infertility.

That tubal disease resulting from a ruptured appendix in childhood should preclude a healthy pregnancy when in vitro fertilization (IVF) is available to bypass this block is as unthinkable as not setting a broken arm. Denying a pregnancy to a patient with Polycystic Ovary Syndrome (PCOS) and ovulatory infertility is as unjust as denying insulin to a diabetic. To not assist fertilization for a man with a low sperm count is as wrong as not intervening in a cardiac arrest.

Another portion of the blame for lack of adequate insurance reimbursement for infertility must rest with the infertility industry, which is generally strongly opposed to mandated coverage. Nothing spends like cash, and collectively we professionals might argue why should we allot considerable resources in billing insurance companies only to receive less money for our services? Too often physician reimbursement is only a small fraction of the charges and is so low as to not even meet the basic operating expenses of a clinic.

With universal insurance coverage for infertility, the inefficiency in care might even worsen with an increase in unnecessary testing, less/more aggressive therapy, and the prolonging of treatment, and in the final analysis lower quality of care. No professional ever believes he or she is overpaid, but is there justification for fertility specialists to be one of the highest paid groups of subspecialists in the United States?

Be assured, the vast majority of physicians are dedicated to their patients and their success, but the fact remains that infertility is big business. A pregnancy is a great product to offer and one on which a price cannot be placed. Unfortunately, this translates to many clinics predominantly treating individuals with high net worth, or those willing and able to incur significant personal debt, never fully appreciating the number of patients who cannot afford to enter their clinic door or who have to stop short of success due to financial restraints. It is estimated that half of infertile couples never seek care, and a portion of the reason is the perceived cost of therapy.

There is a common belief that infertility therapy is expensive; one that hits home when one is reaching into his or her own pocket for each office visit, test, or procedure. In comparison, an IVF cycle may be no more expensive than an emergency room visit with a broken arm or a gall bladder removal. Considerable infertility therapy can be had for less than the cost of breast or dental implants. But then there is no comparison. How can a price be placed on successful infertility therapy, a newborn child? So we must address the central issue of fertility therapy—its efficiency.

Angie Best-Boss and Evelina Weidman Sterling, PhD, are veteran medical writers and women's health advocates. They present a comprehensive overview of the minefield of infertility. There are many books on infertility, but an area that has largely been ignored has been the financial aspects of fertility treatment. Their book bridges this gap. Their insight not only could save you thousands of dollars, it may make that difference in achieving your primary objective—a healthy baby.

Sam Thatcher, MD, PhD
Center for Applied Reproductive Science
Johnson City, TN
May 2008

Introduction:

The Baby Quest

We are definitely both take-charge kind of women, self-proclaimed control freaks—and proud of it! We like to deal with problems head-on—no excuses, no whining, and accepting nothing but the goal. We live by the motto "Don't dwell on the problem, just create a solution." But that was before infertility. Suddenly, for the first time in our lives, we were up against something that couldn't be fixed by hard work alone.

The worst thing about the infertility battle is how powerless you become. You are suddenly no longer in charge of when you will have children. We all have friends who carefully plan their pregnancies so they can deliver their babies without interfering with work deadlines, vacations, or other social plans. When you are experiencing infertility, you can't even choose in which year you have a baby. Infertility touches all aspects of your life—physical, emotional, spiritual, social, and of course, financial. Getting a grip on your finances is one of the few things you can do to regain control of this process.

Determining what you can afford may drive the decisions you make and, ultimately, the course of fertility treatment you choose. By creating a financial plan, you'll make more informed choices and reduce stress. And research shows less emotional stress is a very good thing, perhaps even leading to more fertile moms!

When we started our infertility journeys, we had no idea just how much everything was going to cost. It was easy to avoid dealing with the expenses at first because the initial costs were relatively minor—$50 here and $75 there. (And that doesn't include the hundreds of dollars we spent on the instruments of the devil himself, also known as home pregnancy tests.) And while we were fortunate enough to be able to avoid higher-priced treatments like IVF (in vitro fertilization), we were still shocked at how quickly the out-of-pocket costs added up. And this escalated even more when we both wanted to try again for another child.

After many unexpected turns, a little wiser and with a lot less money in the bank than when we began, we decided we wanted to do something to help others in similar circumstances.

We have spent the last several years involved in helping men and women cope with the difficult path of infertility. This book was born from our journey. One of the most common stories we hear as we meet and work with infertile couples is that understanding and navigating the financial aspect of infertility treatment is overwhelming. It adds a tremendous burden to what is already a difficult time.

This is the only book available to help you understand the nuts and bolts of financing your family building, including: how fertility clinics work, how you can save money on all aspects of your care, and how to maximize your insurance benefits to your advantage. Armed with this resource, you are better prepared to build your family.

We continue to be awed and amazed at the men and women who go to extraordinary lengths to welcome a child into their families. The stamina, dedication, and sheer strength it takes to get through agonizing months and even years of treatment is incredible. Our sincere hope is that by taking charge of your situation and becoming your own best advocate, you will help your own dreams come true.

CHAPTER 1

It Costs *How* Much?:
Make a Fertility Budget Before You Begin

"Like many newly married couples, we had a vision of what our future was going to hold. We had an idealized picture of summer barbeques, holidays surrounded by friends and family, and the sounds of children's laughter filling our home.

"I remember sitting in the doctor's office as he discussed the options, and with each word, those dreams and plans were being taken away from us. Compounding the issue of our diagnosis was the financial obstacles. We were faced with concerns from family and friends, assertions from doctors, and decisions and sacrifices to make."

—JENNA

THE DESIRE TO HAVE A baby is one of the most powerful forces in life, but for one in six couples, having a baby is no easy task. No one ever dreams of having to pay to get pregnant. It may be small comfort, but if you are struggling to conceive, you are not alone. According to the American Society for Reproductive Medicine (ASRM), more than 7.3 million women in the United States have difficulty getting pregnant or carrying a pregnancy to term. While infertility does not discriminate with regard to gender, ethnicity, religion, education, income level, lifestyle, or even family size, access to effective infertility treatment is often grossly unequal.

Infertility is a medical condition with a variety of effective treatment options. With appropriate diagnosis and treatment, nearly 90 percent of individuals struggling to become pregnant are able to bring home a baby. But many women are surprised to find that the costs for the medical treatments necessary to get pregnant are much more expensive than they'd originally planned for.

Several factors can place an undue financial burden on patients, but the most important cause is that infertility treatments are not usually covered by insurance. Some insurance plans cover a few of the expenses related to infertility testing and/or treatment, but most people (more than 70 percent) should expect to pay for the bulk of these costs out of pocket. Given failed IVF cycles, repeat attempts at treatment, and trying for additional children, the overall costs get expensive—fast.

The infertility business is a $4 *billion*-a-year industry. As a result, fertility clinics are not required to provide the most cost-effective and streamlined care. After all, waste is profit. If a clinic can get you to come in for one more appointment, one more test, or one more treatment, it earns more money. It's hard to tell if you received a good standard of care or if you just got ripped off.

Cost is a real impediment to treatment. In fact, less than half of the women and couples in the United States who experience infertility seek help from a doctor. Of those seeking treatment, about half become pregnant using treatments costing between $1,000 and $5,000 per cycle. While this isn't cheap, it's a relative bargain compared to the costs many other families face. Once you start with assisted reproductive therapies (ARTs) like IVF, expect to spend an average of $12,000 per cycle. Because many women don't become pregnant in one cycle, average costs per baby can easily range from $38,000 to $85,000—or even more in some cases.

For some, the path to parenthood is straightforward and short. For others, the road is long and rocky. For all, infertility takes its toll on time, energy, emotions, and finances. The good news is that you have a great chance of becoming pregnant, but be prepared to plan and be involved with all aspects of your infertility care. You will have many tough decisions to make throughout the process, so you need to fully understand your choices and their related consequences. In some cases, you will need to stand your ground, while other circumstances will require a great deal of flexibility.

As with all important money-related decisions, it's critical to start thinking ahead. You have already made an important step by picking up this book. First in this chapter, we're going to talk you through the typical costs for the various forms of fertility treatment that are available to you. Then we'll start to create a financial plan to help you determine how much money you have available to you for this process. In the rest of the book we'll investigate ways to cut the costs of the treatment, so you can be an informed consumer of your health care just as you would be with any other expense in your life. Regardless of your own personal financial situation, we will show you how to get the best quality care for your dollar. You can bring home that beautiful bundle of joy without going broke.

How Much Do Different Treatments Cost?

"At the beginning, the expenses were merely irritating. Since we had no previous experience with infertility, we assumed they were reasonable. Both my husband and I were working and had no children yet, so we expected that the procedures we were paying for would have results and eventually pay off. After eight months of no success and another miscarriage, my doc suggested IVF. By this point we were spent. We had no idea infertility would be so expensive, invasive, and medically affecting as it was. In hindsight, I think there was a lot we could have done to prepare ourselves better."

—TINA

How much does it cost to get pregnant? It depends on many things—age, cause of infertility, your and your partner's general health, your doctor's skills . . . even good old-fashioned luck. What's the short answer? Once you open the door marked "Fertility Treatment," getting pregnant will cost more than you expect.

Just because you are beginning infertility treatment doesn't necessarily mean you are going to undergo a $20,000 procedure. You have a lot of power and resources that can affect your course of treatment. With the right knowledge and skills, you can positively influence both your overall experience and ultimate outcome. First, let's focus on the basic progression of your baby-making journey starting from the very beginning.

PRECONCEPTION PLANNING

Most of us entered adulthood thinking we could have a baby whenever we wanted. The reality is that, biologically speaking, it is amazing anyone gets pregnant. Conception results from a complex chain of events. A woman must first release an egg from her ovaries, the egg must travel through the fallopian tubes toward her uterus, and a man's sperm must join with the egg for fertilization to occur. Finally, the fertilized egg must implant itself into the uterus. Of course, next the embryo needs to grow. Infertility can result from problems that interfere with any of these steps.

Educate yourself about fertility. This can be done through doing your own research and through regular conversations with your gynecologist or other primary care physician (PCP). Don't be afraid to bring the topic up (multiple times if you have to) and talk openly about your family-building plans and concerns. There is no such thing as a stupid question. Your doctor can help you understand your fertility and address any problems as soon as possible.

As we will discuss in more detail in chapter 2, age is a huge factor for women trying to get pregnant. While infertility can strike at any age, with age comes decreasing fertility. The younger you are, the more fertility options you have and the greater the chances for success. If you want to have a baby, trying at thirty or thirty-five is more effective than waiting until after forty. Advanced age is not an impossible obstacle to overcome, but it may well include more time, more money, and more complications—so it's important to plan accordingly.

Recognize, too, that lifestyle factors can affect fertility. Being unhealthy, including being overweight or smoking, can also decrease your fertility. If you want to get pregnant, it's never too early to start focusing on these issues and trying to get yourself as healthy as possible. Sometimes losing a little weight, stopping smoking, or adopting a more health-focused lifestyle can allow you to become pregnant without any further interventions.

INITIAL EVALUATION AND THERAPY

When do you seek help? You may be considered to have impaired fertility if pregnancy has not occurred after one year of unprotected, well-timed intercourse. If you are a woman over thirty-five and have been trying unsuccessfully for over six months, you should consult your gynecologist. Your gynecologist can offer initial testing and information but may then recommend you see a fertility specialist known as a reproductive endocrinologist.

Routine infertility testing will be conducted, including a semen analysis for the male partner and hormone testing and an ultrasound of the female's reproductive organs. Initial treatments will probably include a prescription for fertility medications. This is often coupled with an intrauterine insemination (IUI) where either your partner's sperm or sperm from a donor is placed directly inside your uterus using a small catheter. The good news is that many women become pregnant with these measures, which can cost as little as a few hundred to a few thousand dollars per attempt.

INTERMEDIATE TESTING AND THERAPY

If still nothing is happening, then it's time to try another tactic. More extensive testing will be recommended to assess your reproductive organs in more detail. Most likely, your fertility specialist will be looking for any problems that are prohibiting sperm and egg from meeting. For example, fibroids or endometriosis may be blocking your tubes. If this is found to be the case, your doctor could recommend minor outpatient surgery to check out your uterus and fallopian tubes as well as open up any blockages. Because this is surgery, this will most likely be covered by insurance. Testing and surgery can add thousands to your cost, but probably not out of pocket.

ADVANCED REPRODUCTIVE TECHNOLOGY (ART)

If the sperm and egg are meeting without fertilization or if any blockages cannot be cleared through surgery, in vitro fertilization (IVF) will be considered. With IVF, the doctor is able to facilitate fertilization by putting the eggs and sperm together in a lab. Once fertilization has occurred, your fertility specialist will place the growing embryo into your uterus.

IVF is no longer considered a high-tech or experimental treatment. The first successful IVF cycle was performed in 1978, resulting in the birth of Louise Brown. Since then, more than 1 million babies have been born through IVF worldwide. More than 70,000 cycles of IVF are performed each year in the United States alone. Today, IVF is often combined with intracytoplasmic sperm injection (ICSI), which allows a single sperm to be directly injected into the egg with a small needle in order to maximize fertilization. IVF is expensive (the average cost ranges between $6,000 and

$25,000 per cycle), but success rates are encouraging, with about 40 percent of women bringing home a baby.

Third-Party Reproduction

Third-party reproduction (also known as collaborative reproduction, or surrogate reproduction) is used only as a last resort. Third-party reproduction includes egg donation, embryo donation, sperm donation, and traditional surrogates/gestational carriers. For families who have tried previous options without success, or for families who know from the beginning that they are unable to use their own eggs or uterus, third-party reproduction offers promising hope. Because fertile women are enlisted as donors, surrogates, or gestational carriers, success rates for these treatments are significantly higher—although they are also much more expensive, usually topping $30,000 to $60,000.

IMPORTANT TREATMENT TERMS

ART (Assisted [or Advanced] Reproductive Technology): ART procedures involve surgically removing eggs from a woman's ovaries, combining them with sperm in the laboratory, and returning them to the woman's body or donating them to another woman.

Egg Donation: Donation of an ovum (egg) by one woman to another who attempts to become pregnant by in vitro fertilization (IVF).

Embryo Donation: Rather than destroy the embryos originally created through ART by an infertile couple or donate them to science after that couple completes their family building, the parents decide to donate their frozen embryos to another infertile couple in hopes of giving them a chance at parenthood.

Frozen Embryo Transfer (FET): FET involves IVF with an embryo that has been frozen or cryopreserved.

Gestational Carrier (Gestational Surrogacy): A woman who is not the genetic parent of the baby carries the pregnancy to term. Eggs are extracted from the intended mother or egg donor and mixed with sperm from the intended father or sperm donor in vitro. The embryos are then transferred into the surrogate's uterus.

ICSI (intracytoplasmic sperm injection): A laboratory procedure in which a single sperm is injected directly into an egg; this procedure is most commonly used to overcome male infertility problems.

IUI (intrauterine insemination): A medical procedure in which sperm is placed directly into a woman's uterus to facilitate fertilization (formerly called artificial insemination).

IVF (in vitro fertilization): An ART procedure in which eggs are removed from a woman's ovaries and fertilized outside her body. The resulting embryos are then transferred into the woman's uterus through the cervix.

PGD (Preimplantation Genetic Diagnosis): PGD is a technique that can be used during in vitro fertilization (IVF). After removing a single cell from each embryo, embryos are tested for a variety of genetic disorders. PGD testing is done in the laboratory before the embryo is transferred to the uterus.

Sperm Donation: The practice by which a man donates his sperm to be used by a woman or a couple to achieve a pregnancy.

Traditional Surrogacy: The surrogate mother is artificially inseminated with the sperm of the intended father or sperm donor. The surrogate's own egg is used, thus she will be the genetic mother of the child she is carrying for another family.

The Hidden Costs of Infertility Treatments

"I wish they had a cot for me at the fertility clinic. I get up at 5:00 a.m. to shower and drive thirty minutes away to be at the clinic by 6:30 so I can be first to see the fertility specialist when he comes in at 7:00, because I need to leave by 7:15 to get to work an hour away from the fertility clinic by 8:30 a.m. The driving alone costs an extra $200 a month!"

—SALLY

In addition to the infertility treatments themselves, there are the indirect costs involved—consider everything from lost wages to unexpected medical complications to travel costs. Direct nonmedical expenses can vary and are dependent on how close you are to a reproductive center. These nonmedical costs can be substantial, particularly for highly specialized procedures. Travel expenses such as gas, meals, and lodging can add up, as can other costs such as missed work or lost wages.

Did we mention the hormones? Besides feeling like a pincushion, you may experience the medications' side effects, which can include severe bleeding, lightheadedness, headaches, and nausea. Depending on your reactions and responsibilities, it may affect your ability to maintain your normal work schedule. Plus, all these medical appointments take up a lot of time—many women say that their infertility treatments feel like a part-time job in itself! You have to be at the clinic first thing in the morning for blood work and ultrasounds, and you won't be able to plan more than a day or so in advance of when your eggs will be ripe and ready to start your retrieval or insemination procedure.

With some infertility treatments, there is a higher chance of complications during pregnancy or childbirth, such as preterm labor. You will have a higher chance of multiple births, which further complicates the pregnancy and can lead to long stays for babies in the neonatal intensive care unit. Depending on your insurance coverage and deductibles, you might be responsible for more than you think.

And if you are successful, it's never too soon to think about what you plan to do in the future in terms of growing your family, especially if you have already spent a small fortune on just trying to become pregnant. Is your ultimate goal two children? If so, how does that factor into your decision-making process?

Your Fertility Financial Plan

Because there is no way to predict how long it will take you to get pregnant or exactly what it will involve, *before* you begin the process, you need to determine how much money you can realistically afford to spend on family building. We know, we know—easier said than done, particularly since money is the last thing you want to think about right now. But here's why this is so important: "A lot of people drop out of care and don't end up with their family primarily because they weren't able to plan in advance how they were going to spend their money to end up getting a baby," says

Dr. G. David Adamson, Director of Fertility Physicians of Northern California. "What couples should do is look at all the different choices and decide how much time, how much money, how much emotional energy they are prepared to spend on each one of these choices."

Before you call the closest fertility clinic, you must create a financial plan. A financial plan is a road map that helps you stay on course to reach your financial goals. A sound financial plan is a comprehensive outline dealing with a variety of goals such as retirement, educational funding, insurance, cash flow, tax liabilities, and estate planning, explains Gary A. Howard, an attorney and certified financial planner. "A financial plan includes specific ways to achieve financial goals, and the rationale for the plan. Because a goal can be achieved in many ways, a well-thought-out analysis may include alternative, or 'what if,' scenarios along with the pros and cons of each option."

Your path through infertility may look very different from your best friend's. You have different problems, different resources, different insurance policies, and (hopefully) a different partner! Creating your plan means not just deciding how far you can go financially, but reviewing your emotional, spiritual, and physical limits as well. Your decisions will have long-term effects and need to align with your personal value system. With your partner, if applicable, start the process of creating your own fertility plan.

- **Think about your timeline.** How long are you willing to try on your own before moving on to a fertility specialist? How does age affect your treatment decisions?
- **Think about your own values.** How do you feel about infertility treatments? How does each type fit with your personal and religious beliefs? Do you and your partner agree? What type of emotional toll will these decisions have on you and your partner?
- **Think about your treatment options.** How far do you think you want to go? Are there any treatments that you would be unwilling to try? How will you know if you need to reconsider your original plan? How will you communicate any changes in plan to your partner?
- **Think about limits.** How many cycles are you willing to try? How many cycles can you afford? How will you know if you need

to move on to another option? What options are acceptable to you?

- **Think about your finances.** What is (or isn't) covered by your health insurance? How will you pay for treatments? Do you have a monthly or yearly limit on how much you can spend on treatment? Do you have friends or family who can help out?

"It wasn't until I began to crunch the numbers that I realized we had been living pretty much paycheck to paycheck for the past several years. Oh, we both had good jobs. And we had plenty of money for all the bills and then some, but we hadn't exactly saved anything, nothing substantial anyway. When we found out we needed to undergo IVF, we had to come up with several thousand dollars within a few weeks in order to get started. I guess I always assumed we had more money than we actually did."
—JULIE

You may suddenly find you need to cut down on your basic expenses and start putting money aside specifically for your baby quest. (Refer to the appendices for helpful information on how to create a budget and spending plan.)

If you want take control of your finances, it is essential you make a budget. A budget allows you to get a handle on the flow of your money—how much is coming in and where it goes out. Once you have that information, you can make intelligent choices about how to spend. Inevitably, every person's budget will be different, but there are some basic guidelines that everyone should follow.

The first step in making a realistic budget is figuring out how much money you have coming in. You need to add up your monthly income. On a blank sheet of paper, list the jobs for which you receive a salary or wages. Then, list all self-employment for which you receive income, including farm income and sales commissions. If you are in a salaried position, simply divide your yearly income by 12. Finally, list other sources of income, such as child support or bonuses.

Next, you'll need to know where your money goes during a set period. While some expenses remain constant and are easy to figure out (rent, car insurance, car payments, phone and cable bills), other expenses such as utilities, gas, food, and entertainment may change from month to month. The best way to figure them into your budget is to come up with a monthly average for each one.

By looking at your spending, you can make special note of any nonessential spending that you may be doing and make cuts as necessary.

> *"I admit it . . . merely keeping tabs on every expense is enough to make anyone spend less. If I have to 'fess up to the number of trips I make to Starbucks a week, I get a little squeamish. But I want to have enough money to do whatever we need to get a baby, but I didn't realize how much money I wasted, particularly when I'm feeling blue."*
>
> —JILL

Many financial planners suggest living by the 60 Percent Rule. The basic idea is that all your "essential" spending—taxes, food, shelter, clothing and the rest—comes out of the first 60 percent of your total, pretax income. The rest, in 10 percent chunks, is devoted to retirement savings, emergency savings (or debt repayment), short-term savings for irregular expenses (like holidays and car repairs), and fun money.

Add up your essentials. You may not spend more than that percentage of your income. That's nonnegotiable. Your wiggle room is in the other 40 percent. Your infertility expenses may take up more than 10 percent, but they cannot take up more than you need for essentials.

This is only the beginning of a long journey of maintaining financial health for your family. If you're going to stop working after your baby arrives, now is the time to start practicing living on less. The same goes if you're going to take an unpaid maternity leave, even if it will only be temporary. If you aren't covered by disability insurance, get it now, since you won't be able to once you become pregnant.

Focus on both your short-term and long-term goals. "Funding the costs of infertility treatments or adoption are for the most part short-term financial goals. Long-term goals include retirement, appropriate and affordable insurance protection, maintaining adequate cash reserves, and minimizing consumer credit card debt. Comprehensive financial planning encompasses a variety of goals and priorities," says Howard.

Once you know how much you have to work with, start evaluating which infertility treatments best fit with your budget and are most realistic for you and your family.

Money and Your Relationship

Dueling over dollars is a common problem in marriage—and a common cause for divorce. If you don't take the time to talk about money, it could end up taking a major toll on your relationship. Money is a leading cause of marital strife. Pile on the stress of going through infertility, and this is a disaster waiting to happen.

When considering your finances, look for underlying issues. Perhaps there are other problems going on, such as concerns about security and control. Or maybe the impending overwhelming responsibility of becoming a parent is adding to the stress levels. Rather than becoming irritated with your partner, recognize that arguments over money may indicate other problems as well.

Realize that both partners must be involved with the decision-making about money and how to pay for family-building options. And understand that you both may have different money styles. You may view money differently, so you will need to talk openly about how you think about money and how it should be spent. Always listen to your partner. A key to developing a good financial plan is having both of you fully involved at each step.

Establish some ground rules about your money. You will need to set some boundaries so you both feel in control of your financial future, especially how it pertains to growing your family. Compromise is a necessity. You will need to set your financial goals together. This includes the short-term family building goals as well as the longer-term plans as to what you will do after your child or children arrive.

Together draft a budget and cash-flow statement. "It's like going on a diet," says Victoria Collins, financial planner, psychologist, and author of *Couples and Money: A Couple's Guide Updated for the New Millennium.* "You hate to step on the scale, but if you come up with a concrete action plan, it's easier to follow through."

"Put it on paper," she advises. "Just having an agreement helps."

If money is a problem now, the financial stress is not going to go away once you have succeeded in building your family. Money doesn't have to ruin your marriage. Instead, it can strengthen the bond by teaching you how to work as partners. What might have once torn you and your partner apart can actually bring you together as you work toward a common goal.

Weigh Your Options

"We took out a loan to start the IVF process for the first time, and my son will be six years old this winter; we just paid for him in full last year. Every day I look at him and see our very own miracle. I also have a seven-month-old, thanks again to IVF and our miracle worker doctors. This time we were lucky enough to get pregnant on our first try. When you look into their eyes for the first time, the money, shots, stress, tears, all the not-so-fun stuff is forgotten. Some people have expensive trucks and vacation cruises . . . we have Corey and Kate."

—Stephanie

Infertility will affect you in ways you never imagined—from trying to come up with cash as fast as possible to completely losing your sense of privacy and modesty to feeling emotionally drained for months or years on end. These raw feelings and emotions can be overwhelming. As you can, maintain a sense of composure and control, believing you will make it through! The more active you are in conscious decision making, the better off you will be in both the short term and the long term.

Now is the time to start thinking about these complex issues. If you're reading this book, you're well on your way to trying to make a baby. As uncomfortable as it can be, you and your partner must sit down and closely examine your goals and finances. The last thing you want to do is to welcome a baby into your home with no money and worries about how you are going to pay the bills.

No one wants to put a limit on how much they will spend on a baby. But you need to think carefully about this or you will get caught up in the vicious cycle of making a baby and not realize how much you are actually spending. Before you know it, you could be deep in debt with fewer options and an unforeseen impact on your future ability to raise and educate the children who come into your family. Keep track of your goals and prepare carefully for your decisions. It's never too early to think ahead. Ask yourself:

- Should you get pregnant and give birth, how much money will you need to pay for your child's basic needs, for day care, or for potential medical issues the child may experience?
- Should you reserve funds for pursuing other paths to parenthood?
- How many children do you want to have?

For most of us, sacrifices are inevitable. We might suddenly realize we don't have time to waste and must get started trying to have a baby sooner than we would have liked. We might have to give up on Plan A to move to Plan B or Plan C. Some might choose to give up their time and take second jobs to make extra money to spend on family building. Others opt to slash away at any perceived extras in spending to save money. It may seem difficult at first, but keep your eye on the prize: you are investing in your family's future. How far are you willing to go? Ask yourself:

- Are you willing to take out a loan? If so, for how much?
- Are you willing to move to another state or accept a job that offers better fertility benefits?
- Are you willing to sell your nice new car and drive a used model?
- Are you willing to downsize your lifestyle?
- Are you willing to ask friends and family for assistance?
- Are you willing to tap into your savings account or use your retirement money?

> *"As the medical bills swarmed the mailbox, it was crucial we had some tough conversations about what was considered a like-to-have and a need-to-have item. We both traded in our cars to get junkers so we could increase our monthly cash flow. We also cut our food budget in half and went out only on special occasions. Although it felt like punishment at first, it quickly turned to a positive thing. We were both looking to our future."*
>
> —Matt

Planning Your Family's Future

"If you can't afford to have infertility treatments, then how are you going to afford a child? I swear to God, if one more person utters those words in my presence, I may not be responsible for my actions."

—LYNETTE

What does it cost to raise a child? According to the U.S. Department of Agriculture, it's about $165,600. Expenses include housing, food, transportation, clothing, health care, education and child care, and other miscellaneous expenses (personal care items, recreation expenses, et cetera). Costs do not include college expenses or indirect costs (such as a parent taking work leave to raise the child). Kids are expensive—no argument there.

But when you leave the hospital with your baby, nobody is standing at the door demanding a check for $170,000. Or even $25,000 to cover the first few years. That's why paying for infertility is so difficult—you are expected to pay a lot of money up front. You will want to make financially sound decisions so you don't compromise your family's future, but don't let those child-rearing numbers scare you.

Trying for Number Two

"After I miscarried, someone said to me, 'Children are expensive, at least with only one you'll save money.' Unbelievable. I really want a playmate for my daughter. I know she'll enjoy being a big sister. I remember how much fun it was growing up in a big family. But sometimes I worry I must be a horrible mother for investing my energy—and money!—on trying anything possible to have another child that it takes away from my first born."

—LESLIE

What if you already have one child but can't get (or stay) pregnant with number two? Statistically, secondary infertility is more common than primary infertility. While the causes of secondary infertility are often similar to those for primary infertility, second and third babies can be harder to conceive simply due to the passage of time. In other words, your eggs and your partner's sperm are older than they were the last time you tried baby making.

Whether or not it was easy to get pregnant the first time, dealing with secondary infertility is difficult. Besides the physical and emotional toll, trying for another child isn't cheap. Couples often feel guilty about spending so much money trying to conceive a second child when they already have a child on which they could be spending those resources. Is it better for Johnny to have a college account or a baby sister?

Carefully consider the consequences of your financial plan. If either you or your partner want to be a stay-at-home parent, can you afford to do so if you continue to pursue infertility treatment? Look at the long-term consequences for each of your possible options. For example, if you do not try at least one IUI for a second child, will you always have regrets? What if you go into so much debt you spend the next five years living paycheck to paycheck? Will you regret not having enough money for vacations, ice cream out, or even preschool?

And if you're just thinking about number two after having trouble conceiving number one, then seek help early. Remember, the longer you wait, the more it can cost.

Getting Started

Once you decide how much you have to spend on family building, the next decision is how to find the best and most cost-effective medical care. We are going to walk you through all the steps to help you be your own best advocate. We'll give you plenty of valuable advice about how to best prepare yourself for the financial challenges you will encounter. You have a lot to consider, and with appropriate planning, you will be able to have a baby.

Five Things You Can Do Right Now

1. Gather all of your pay stubs and records of other sources of income.
2. List your expenses.
3. Create a budget and commit to living by it.
4. Decide how much money you are willing and able to allocate for family building.
5. Consider how you will divide and allocate your financial resources.

CHAPTER 2

Baby-Making Basics:
Increase Your Chances from the Start

"I never gave any thought to my fertility before, not even for a second. In fact, my parents drilled it into me . . . it only takes one time, Kathie, so be really, really careful. Wow, was I in for a rude awakening! I wish I had asked more questions and got to know my body better before I tried to become pregnant."

—KATHIE

MOST OF US SPEND A lot of time and energy trying to avoid pregnancy, so it is not surprising we don't know what to expect when we are actually trying to make a baby. Only 20 percent of couples actively trying to become pregnant do so in any given month. It's perfectly normal for a young fertile woman to take up to a year to become pregnant.

By getting to know your body, understanding your fertility, and asking the right questions from the beginning, you can dramatically increase your chances of becoming pregnant while saving money.

Preserving Your Fertility

If you want to have a baby, it's never too early to think about your fertility. Things you do (or don't do) now can impact your ability to have a baby later. Everything from undiagnosed sexually transmitted infections to exposure to environmental toxins can affect your ability to make a baby. Taking good care of yourself before you want to get pregnant will help you when you're ready to start trying.

DON'T WAIT TOO LONG
As you consider your family-building options, be aware that age is the most crucial factor affecting your fertility. In today's society, women are waiting

longer to have children. In fact, over 20 percent of women are waiting until after age thirty-five to start a family.

Fertility decreases with age for both men and women. We wish it weren't so, but women are born with a limited number of eggs, and that number and quality of remaining eggs decline over time. Since every woman's body ages at a different rate, there is no way to accurately predict your future fertility. Fertility starts to decline in your twenties, and more dramatically after age thirty-five. For men, aging affects sperm shape and motility (how well they swim). Although fertility treatments can be effective, age affects how you will respond to treatment. Success rates for IVF decrease dramatically for women in their late thirties and forties. It is important that you are informed and seek assistance as soon as possible in order to increase your chances for success.

JUST SAY NO!

There are a few basic but important rules about getting pregnant that we'd be remiss in neglecting to include. It seems like simple stuff, but these factors can play a major role in fertility for both men and women.

- **Don't smoke.** Smoking can negatively impact virtually every aspect of fertility, and some fertility specialists will refuse to treat people who smoke.
- **If you drink, go easy.** Large amounts of alcohol (more than two drinks per day) may lower your odds of parenthood.
- **Don't do drugs.** All recreational and illegal drugs, including marijuana and steroids, can contribute to infertility.
- **Check your medicine cabinet.** Over-the-counter or prescription drugs, including antibiotics, painkillers, antidepressants, and hormonal treatments, can decrease fertility.
- **Be careful with herbal remedies.** Herbal treatments may prove to be beneficial, but never experiment on your own since they can also be very potent. If you are interested in these types of treatment options, consult a trained naturopathic doctor.

EAT RIGHT

- Eat a well-balanced diet full of natural foods, including plenty of fruits and vegetables.

- Avoid foods with caffeine, additives, or any artificial flavorings or colors.
- Up your vitamin C intake, including grapefruits, guavas, oranges, kiwis, mango, and papaya.
- Select foods that have vitamin E, including wheat germ, almonds, sunflower seeds, sunflower oil, safflower oil, hazelnuts, peanuts, peanut butter, spinach, broccoli, corn oil, soybean oil, and fortified cereals.
- Round out your diet with foods rich in zinc, such as red meat, poultry, some seafood, beans, nuts, whole grains, fortified cereals, and dairy products.
- Choose foods with folic acid, such as dark green, leafy vegetables, whole wheat bread, lightly cooked beans and peas, nuts and seeds, sprouts, oranges and grapefruits, liver and other organ meats, poultry, and fortified breakfast cereals and enriched grain products.
- Women should also take a supplement of at least 400 micrograms daily of folic acid to help prevent birth defects.

MAINTAIN A HEALTHY WEIGHT
(FOR BOTH WOMEN AND MEN)

Weight is another important concern. Research has shown that heavier women and men may face more fertility problems. According to the American Society for Reproductive Medicine (ASRM), 12 percent of all infertility cases are a result of either partner weighing either too much or too little. Body weight affects estrogen. If a woman has too much body fat, she will produce too much estrogen, which can cause her not to release eggs. Likewise, if a woman has too little body fat, she can't produce enough estrogen, so her reproductive cycle shuts down. Weight management and good nutrition for both men and women are key elements.

It is important to maintain a body mass index (BMI) of between 19 and 30 while trying to conceive. A BMI between 19 and 25 is ideal. BMI takes into account your optimal weight for your height. To calculate your BMI, visit the CDC website at http://www.cdc.gov/nccdphp/dnpa/bmi/.

Regular exercise is also important while trying to have a baby. But don't overdo it. If you exercise too much or push your body too hard, you might throw your hormones out of whack. Moderation is the key to good fertility. Put training for the marathon on hold.

Although taking good care of yourself and doing all the right things physically and mentally will increase your chances for success, there are no guarantees. Don't take it as a sign of personal failure if you don't get the results you want. Blocked fallopian tubes won't "unblock" no matter how many relaxation exercises you do. Don't waste precious time focusing on lifestyle changes only. See a doctor! Infertility is a disease, which for many requires specific medical treatment.

Know Your Fertility

You can start assessing your fertility at any time without leaving the comfort of your bathroom. A number of at-home tests evaluate your ovulation, whether or not you're pregnant, and even how well your partner's sperm swims. While all the tests work on some level, many are difficult to interpret. Nearly all involve spending money, and some are better than others.

CHARTING OVULATION

The oldest and most low-tech method is to take your basal body temperature (BBT). You can get a special basal body thermometer at any pharmacy

---

YOUR FERTILE PERIOD

Your fertile period is the time during which having sexual intercourse could lead to a pregnancy. When is yours?

Begin counting on the first day of your menstrual period. Women normally ovulate about 14 days from the first day of their period, although this varies considerably from woman to woman. As a result, it is helpful to know exactly when, and if, you ovulate, rather than simply relying on the 14-day rule. You can do this through at-home ovulation monitoring.

In general, your fertile period starts about 4 to 5 days before ovulation, and ends about 24 to 48 hours afterwards because sperm can live in your body for approximately 4 to 7 days, and the egg can live for 24 to 48 hours after being released. You are most fertile a couple of days before ovulation and the day of ovulation. Knowing your fertile days can help you increase your chances of getting pregnant.

for about ten bucks. Get a *specific basal body thermometer*, since it is usually more sensitive to slight temperature changes than a traditional thermometer. Each morning before you get out of bed, take your temperature. You can ask your physician for a special chart to track these changes. Better yet, you can download free, easy-to-use charts from dozens of web pages on the internet. Just type "free BBT chart" into your favorite search engine.

Fertility specialists will expect you to track your cycles. If you haven't already done this, start right away. Bring at least three months' of charts to your appointment. If not, your fertility specialist might very well send you home after your first appointment with a "Let's talk again once you have had time to chart your cycle." This could set you back several months, not to mention the cost of a nonproductive appointment.

WHAT IS A NORMAL CYCLE?

The menstrual cycle is from Day 1 of bleeding to Day 1 of the next time of bleeding. Although the average cycle is 28 days, it is perfectly normal to have a cycle as short as 21 days or as long as 35 days. If your cycles are longer than 35 days, talk to a fertility specialist right away, since this could be affecting your ability to become pregnant. Ovulation occurs almost exactly 14 days prior to the first day of the next menstrual cycle. In other words, if cycles are 30 days apart (from the first day of bleeding of cycle 1 to the first day of bleeding of cycle 2), then ovulation occurs on day 16.

Even without a BBT, your body is giving you all sorts of signs about your ovulation—you just have to know how to translate them!

Many women experience *mittelschmerz,* the midcycle pain associated with ovulation. You may feel crampy and have mild abdominal pain. Many women experience this discomfort as the cyst encapsulating the egg ruptures, releasing the unfertilized egg.

Your cervical fluid will change as you ovulate. The mucus will thin out and become watery (it will resemble an egg white), which helps the sperm travel through the cervix and into the uterus and fallopian tube. The amount of this thin mucus increases right up until ovulation.

Your cervix may change during your cycle as well. During the beginning of your cycle, your cervix is low, hard, and closed. As ovulation takes place, it pulls up, softens, and opens just a bit. You can check with two fingers and track what it feels like.

However, the easiest way to tell if you're ovulating may be your increased libido! Not everybody has these signs, but if you know how to read them, it's more information. In her book *Taking Charge of Your Fertility*, Toni Weschler explains how you can gain better control over your health and life if you take the time to understand your fertility; it's a must-read for any women seeking to get pregnant.

OVULATION PREDICTOR TESTS

For those who don't mind peeing on a stick (something you'd better get used to during your pregnancy quest, if you haven't already!), you can also purchase an ovulation predictor kit (OPK). At $20 for a pack of five, these kits measure the amount of luteinizing hormone (or LH, one of the hormones needed for ovulation) in your urine. The darker the test line, the more LH you have and the more likely you are about to ovulate. Unlike the BBT, the OPK actually lets you know 24 to 48 hours *before* you ovulate, giving you time to have baby-making sex in preparation for, not just in reaction to, your body's optimal fertility time.

The drawbacks? You get only five tests per pack and the shades of the lines can be tough to read. Digital ones are easier to interpret, but they cost about $10 more per package. Plus, if your cycles are quirky, you might get a false reading or not know when to begin testing. And those five tests can go very quickly. Some women we know have used them all up in a single day. (Hey, the light was bad and a lot could happen in twelve hours.) It's not unheard of to go through a couple of packs a month.

Other variables, like drinking too much, testing at the wrong time of day, even medical issues like polycystic ovary syndrome (PCOS), can all affect the reliability of OPKs. So talk to your doctor about how to best use an OPK. It's best to limit yourself to one test per day. Going overboard wastes your money and yanks your emotional chain.

Another ovulation predictor tool is the daily fertility monitor. This instrument is a little pricier—about $200 for the initial monitor and $50 a month for refills. Available in most pharmacies, the fertility monitor is an ovulation predictor that checks the amount of LH in your urine. With the daily fertility monitor, you have to pee on the stick first thing in the morning every single day of the month. Besides being a pain to remember, the fertility monitor is effective only for women with fairly normal and predictable cycles. Since you are already experiencing some sort of infertility issue, this might rule you out. While it's a better choice than hundreds of individual OPKs, it is still expensive.

Other popular at-home fertility monitor options include the saliva ovulation predictor test and the ovulation watch. Each month, your saliva goes through changes as your hormones fluctuate. One of these hormones is estrogen. Just prior to ovulation, estrogen levels increase and create a distinct pattern in your dried saliva that looks like frost on a windowpane. This pattern is called ferning and is visible only under the kit's special microscope, costing between $25 and $50. Most fertility specialists agree this type of ferning pattern is extremely difficult to see and may not be reliable anyway. We don't recommend the saliva ovulation test to budget-conscious mothers-to-be.

The ovulation watch measures the numerous salts (chloride, sodium, potassium) in a woman's sweat, which also change during the menstrual cycle. A big benefit is that the ovulation watch detects the salt surge five days *prior* to ovulation. Worn while sleeping, the ovulation watch makes an earlier predictor of ovulation than any other chemical surge during the month. As a result, this watch has gotten rave reviews, but the price is still very steep. At $200 for the watch and another $50 per month for the special salt-measuring sensors, it's a fun toy, but it's too much money for too little benefit.

The bottom line? Save your money, chart your BBT, learn more about other ovulation signs, and have sex every other day from day 10 to day 21 to be safe.

FERTILITY TESTING

For those with money to burn, over-the-counter fertility testing kits claim to evaluate key fertility elements. These at-home fertility tests include tests for men and women and can be yours for around $100. The male test measures the concentration of motile sperm, but it ignores two other important healthy sperm factors: sperm count and morphology. The female test detects follicle stimulating hormone (FSH) on Day 3 of the menstrual cycle, but since a woman's levels fluctuate widely, this test is virtually useless. One company salesman even admitted they added the women's tests only so men wouldn't feel bad about having to test their semen.

Our major concern: you and your partner may be fooled by seemingly good results and wait longer to seek professional medical care. *Don't waste your money or your time.* Buck up and see a real live fertility specialist as soon as you think there might be a problem. All fertility specialists will want to repeat these tests using much more sensitive measures regardless of what these at-home test results say anyway.

The conception-enhancing kits are yet another opportunity to throw away your fertility dollars. While the advertisements suggest they can overcome low sperm counts, low sperm motility, a tilted cervix, and pH imbalances, you are paying $300 for a semen collector (condom) and a single-use cervical cap which, once filled with semen, is supposed to bring the sperm in closer contact with the opening of the uterus. The directions on how to use these items correctly sound intimidating, even to us. Results are going to be no better than well-timed intercourse, explains fertility specialist Dr. Mark Trolice, so that $300 is better spent on a legit infertility treatment. Despite slick marketing tactics, these kits are not a treatment for infertility and do not replace a trip to a fertility clinic.

PREGNANCY TESTS

As you well know, there are myriad home pregnancy tests, and these have become increasingly effective in recent years. But be careful: you can easily rack up the bucks buying these tests in bulk. (We know, we know, this time you might actually be pregnant.) Taking at-home pregnancy tests is fine, but look out for your pocketbook.

Pregnancy tests run about $10 to $20 a pop. At first glance, this seems like a relatively cheap answer to the million-dollar question, Am I pregnant? But we know women who have bought them in bulk—by the hundreds. Seriously. Do the math—it adds up!

"Ah, the pee stick aisle in the market. I know it well. It's as much an addiction as anything else. I had to sneak them in the house to pee

on them, much like someone with a drinking or drug habit would
have to do it in secret. No one in my life understood this compulsion
I had to take those pregnancy tests."

—GILLIAN

If your boobs hurt so much you can't wear a shirt, or if you suddenly wake up several times a night to pee, or if the smell of something as innocuous as toast makes you want to hurl, then go for it and spring for a test. If not, try really, really hard to remain calm. At the very least, wait a full two weeks after you think you have ovulated before you become obsessive. Doing a pregnancy test any earlier just isn't going to bring you the news you want. If you can't fight the temptation any longer, go for the cheapies. Dollar stores sell tests that work; they all measure the level of HCG, a pregnancy hormone. No matter how much wishful thinking you do, a more expensive test isn't going to make you pregnant.

BABY-MAKING SEX

Having sex on a schedule can be frustrating and intimidating. Still, enjoy your time together and don't forget the romance. A few helpful hints to maximize your fertility:

- Go natural—don't use lotions, saliva, or lubricants, since they slow down or kill the sperm. If you have to use something, try the so-called fertility-friendly lubes, which are water-based.
- Don't douche, since it will wash out the sperm.
- The best position is the traditional missionary style (meaning man on top), because it puts the sperm as close to the cervix as possible.
- Make love at least every other day during your fertile time (2 to 3 days before *and* after ovulation).
- If possible, remain still for about 20 to 30 minutes after sex in order to provide more time for the sperm to find its way into your uterus. A pillow under your hips doesn't hurt either, but a regular pillow does just fine. Do not waste your money on the $140 fertility pillow!
- Relax and have fun!

Patience Is a Virtue

It's hard to be patient. We want to know what's wrong and how to fix it right now. But a word of caution: companies are lining up to take advantage of you. Many of these products will not provide you with enough useful information to make it worth your time and money, and the costs add up quickly. Get to know your body the natural way, and in general that means staying far, far away from the "pregnancy and fertility" aisle at your local pharmacy. Instead, save your pennies and spend your hard-earned money on something with more of a potential impact—like testing and treatments with a doctor. If you must try one of these infertility trinkets, check eBay to find them at a much lower cost.

Your Gynecologist's Office

You might have suspected for some time that everything might not be so rosy in the baby-making department. The women in your family have had trouble getting pregnant, your periods have always been irregular or have even been known to take a leave of absence for no good reason. For others, it might be the gynecologist who first identifies something unusual in a routine lab test or exam that suggests getting pregnant will be a little more difficult. In fact, discussion about your fertility should always be a part of your yearly exam. Whatever your situation, the gynecologist's office is usually the first stop on the journey to have a baby.

Your gynecologist and your primary care physician (PCP) can be good initial resources. Once you realize there might be more to baby making than you expected, take advantage of all your gynecologist and PCP have to offer. Often gynecologists just concentrate on your pelvic region, but your general health plays an important role in baby making as well. Talk about your overall health and preconception concerns.

Both you and your partner need to undergo a complete physical to rule out any obvious underlying causes of infertility and ensure you are in the best possible physical shape to move forward. Now is also the time to address general health-related issues, such as smoking, drinking, exercise, diet, or weight, since all of these can negatively impact your chances of having a baby. While you are at it, confirm you are up-to-date on your vaccinations, since some illnesses can contribute to infertility or cause you to miscarry. Your gynecologist can go a step further and do a lot of the very basic tests associated with the infertility diagnosis: hormone testing, sexually transmitted infection testing, and even an ultrasound to check out your ovaries and uterine lining. Some gynecologists are even willing to order a semen analysis. Your gynecologist can also help you understand how to track your fertility and recognize your most fertile times.

Periodically (at least once a year or so) ask for copies of any updates on your medical information—reports, tests, everything! Keep these papers and reports in a safe place. You will need these documents again throughout your fertility journey.

The First Line of Defense: Clomiphene Citrate

Unless your gynecologist comes to the conclusion you need to see a specialist right away, he or she might prescribe the medication clomiphene citrate (more commonly known under its trade names Clomid or Serophene). This is a relatively cheap pill (about $10 to $60 for an initial attempt) taken for five days towards the beginning of the menstrual cycle order to promote ovulation. Clomiphene citrate tricks the body into producing more FSH and LH, two hormones needed for ovulation. This helps women produce eggs so they have a higher chance of becoming pregnant. Because of its effectiveness and low cost, it is prescribed routinely by gynecologists as a first-line treatment.

Most important, you must determine if you are actually ovulating on clomiphene citrate, especially if you have hormonal problems like polycystic ovary syndrome, which may inhibit your ability to ovulate. If you aren't ovulating, you can't get pregnant. Just because you get your period does not mean you are ovulating. The only way to know is to continue tracking your ovulation through temperature charting, checking your cervical fluids and additional signs of ovulation, using ovulation predictor tests, and undergoing any lab tests ordered by your doctor.

Age is the most important factor determining the success of clomiphene citrate. As we've said before (and as you'll hear countless times throughout your fertility quest), there is no getting around the fact that fertility declines with age. Thus, clomiphene citrate might not be the best course of action for women in their late thirties or early forties. If it's not effective, you are wasting precious fertile time. Get to a fertility specialist now for a more appropriate treatment plan and more potent medications.

Even if you are ovulating on clomiphene citrate, if you aren't pregnant after a few months you need to move on. You have about a 33 percent chance of becoming pregnant within the first three months of using clomiphene citrate. If you have PCOS, your physician should also prescribe an insulin sensitizer drug like metformin. After four months of ovulatory cycles, you have less than a 10 percent chance of achieving pregnancy, so it isn't worth continuing any longer. Staying on it longer than necessary is one of the most common wastes of fertility time and money.

Moving On

Don't get waylaid for too long at the gynecologist's office. Gynecologists have a bad reputation for saying you have plenty of time to get pregnant and not to worry. As a result, they may be slow to suggest seeing a fertility specialist, even though there's only so much a gynecologist can do. Look at it this way: When we have something go wrong with our house, most of us call our neighborhood handyman to check things out. He will usually do some simple diagnostics to find the root of the problem. If it turns out to be something major with the electrical system, we don't risk our house burning down by calling the jack-of-all-trades handyman (no matter how much we like him and are impressed with his work). We call a professional, certified, insured, and bonded master electrician from a reputable company—a specialist.

The same can be said for moving on to a fertility specialist after your initial consultations with your gynecologist. Your gynecologist knows the basics but isn't a specialist. Between Pap smears, yeast infections, sexually transmitted infections, and delivering babies in the middle of the night, your fertility may not be his or her top priority. If you feel it's been too long with no results, you need to move forward.

In the next chapter, we'll give you tips for finding the best fertility specialist and working with him or her to create a treatment plan to get you pregnant.

Five Things You Can Do Right Now

1. Collect all of your medical records for yourself and your partner.
2. Begin charting your cycle now.
3. Schedule a checkup with your GYN if you haven't done so in the last six months.
4. Evaluate your and your partner's health and lifestyle and make healthy changes.
5. Begin exercising moderately and eating well if you do not do so already.

Chapter 3

Finding the Best Care:
Select a Fertility Clinic

"I was on the phone with my gynecologist when I first heard the words reproductive endocrinologist. He gave me the phone numbers for a few specialists who could handle my case beyond the standard basal body temperature chart and multiple rounds of Clomid therapy. In the end, we went with the closest and cheapest option. Unfortunately, this ended up being entirely the wrong decision for us."

—Lisa

Congratulations! You have made the scary yet critical decision to move on to more specialized care in your baby quest. Now what? Let your fingers do the walking and flip through the yellow pages? Perhaps, but there are better ways. You have many choices; there are more than nine hundred trained fertility specialists in the United States. Where do you start?

Fertility clinics are not very evenly dispersed throughout the country, meaning that your options may be limited simply due to geography. For a listing of fertility specialists in the United States, you can visit the Society for Reproductive Endocrinology and Infertility (SREI) at www.socrei.org. Clinics are more common around large cities or very populated states, such as Massachusetts, New York, and California. For those who live in more rural and less populated regions, you might not have a fertility clinic in your state. Maine, Wyoming, and Montana all currently have none. If you do not have a fertility clinic close to home, you can either travel to another city or state, or work with a local gynecologist who has significant experience treating infertility. However, a general gynecologist cannot perform any assisted reproductive technologies (ARTs), including IVF, because he or she won't have an appropriate laboratory or laboratory support.

Once you have a list of potential clinics, what's the next step? Not all clinics are created equal. Fertility is big business, and these clinics actively compete for your business. Some spend considerable resources marketing to potential clients, and many large fertility clinics have a full-time professional marketing and public relations staff. These clinics can be impeccably decorated, provide spalike atmospheres with beautiful (and pricey) artwork and waterfalls, and are located in high-end neighborhoods to make themselves very attractive to you, the much desired patient. But beware: the beautiful façade doesn't always translate to the best care.

Clinics also regularly participate in direct advertising through billboards, magazines, newspapers, radio, the internet, and even on television. They each announce unparalleled success rates combined with the newest technology. One clinic even entices potential patients by hosting an all-expense-paid informational dinner at a five-star restaurant complete with goodie bags containing free makeup, gift certificates, and even a new pair of shoes! Be a smart consumer and don't be blinded by the bling.

What's Right for You?

How do you decide which clinic is the best for you? Everyone has different criteria as to what they find most attractive, appealing, or comforting. Whatever your preferences, fully explore your options from the onset. Talk with several clinics before making a final decision. Fertility treatment is a time-consuming, emotionally draining, and very expensive endeavor. You deserve compassionate care. A few important questions to ask your clinic:

- How long has the clinic been in existence?
- How many patients have been treated at the clinic?
- What is the specific training of the medical personnel?
- Can you receive written material about the clinic and the procedures it offers?

Get Recommendations

There are strategic ways to determine which clinic is the best for you, but it takes research and homework. Thoroughly investigate the clinics. One of the easiest and quickest ways to gather information about potential clinics is to talk to your close friends and/or health care providers.

Once you start talking, you may be surprised to learn how many others have very similar experiences and might even have some helpful stories and advice to share. You also can go online to infertility bulletin boards and blogs. Every clinic will have supporters and detractors, but you can learn a lot about the inner workings of clinics by talking with other patients, both in person and in cyberspace. Online infertility bulletin boards abound, and many people are gracious and willing to share their experiences and suggestions.

Talk to medical professionals you know and trust. Not only do these medical professionals maintain relationships with their colleagues, but there is a good chance they (or someone close to them) went through infertility as well. Since infertility is not a banner proudly displayed, you may never know others' experiences until you start talking openly.

Infertility magazines, advocacy groups, and organizations routinely publish lists of "recommended" fertility clinics and physicians. "These are top-notch doctors," says one group's spokesperson. Maybe, but roughly translated, these doctors have paid to become professional members, have bought advertisements, or have made a donation to the organization. Often, these sponsored "best of" lists are biased, although you may like knowing that these doctors support an organization that supports infertility patients.

Other for-profit agencies and companies promise to screen doctors for you. Popular professional physician-matching websites typically charge doctors a hefty $3,000 just to get on their online referral list. If your doctor is so hard-up for clients he or she needs to pay to be on a list, we'd be wary.

Finding the right specialist isn't an exact science, and you will have to rely on a combination of factors to find the best fit for you. All of this information can help you develop your short list of potential candidates.

Just How Good Is My Clinic?: The Truth About Statistics

You want the clinic that does the best job of getting people pregnant. How hard can it be? All fertility clinics get people pregnant, but some are better at it than others. How can you tell just how good they are?

The Fertility Clinic Success Rate and Certification Act of 1992 requires that all U.S. fertility clinics performing ARTs report success rates to the Centers for Disease Control and Prevention (CDC). While this is a federal requirement, there is no penalty for clinics that refuse to participate. Fertility clinics are also encouraged to become members of the Society for Assisted Reproductive Technology (SART) and submit their statistics each year to them as well. However, some clinics don't want to pay the required membership fees to belong to SART.

Most clinics gladly supply their numbers for peer and patient review through the CDC or SART, but a handful of clinics still refuse to report their statistics. Some argue the reporting process is flawed and they therefore won't participate. And it is an imperfect system—no argument there. But the numbers still can be useful to patients in making their decisions. For those who don't follow the CDC's reporting guidelines, consider why they aren't doing so. It could mean they had a bad year and don't want to report those statistics and blemish an otherwise stellar reputation. Or, it could imply they don't play well with their peers and aren't interested in empowering you as a patient. Whatever the reason, be cautious about clinics that don't report. Where do you find a clinic's statistics? ART statistical reports can be accessed at www.cdc.gov and www.sart.org.

Deconstructing a Report

Statistics can provide some valuable insight into the internal workings of the clinic and help you gain a better overview of the success rates of the clinics you are considering. On pages 37–39 you can find a sample report as well as a description of each section. Report sections include:

Types of ART

It is important to look at number and types of ART cycles performed, which can include some combination of IVF, ICSI, GIFT, and ZIFT. Not all clinics offer the same services, and the number of ART procedures vary from just a handful to hundreds per year. In the sample report, all of the cycles were IVF, which is fairly typical now. Any clinic performing fewer than 25 IVF cycles per year should be carefully scrutinized, as it may not have the experience you need.

Procedural Factors

This is where specialized procedures like ICSI during the IVF cycle or surrogacy attempts are listed. Unstimulated cycles mean no medications were used. If you have a particular concern, such as male factor infertility and know, for example, that ICSI is going to be necessary, you will want a clinic that does it routinely. Still, you may not want a clinic that reports an unusually high percentage of specialized procedures, since it may be inclined to pressure you into something you don't want or need. In the sample report, 40 percent of IVF cycles involved ICSI.

Patient Diagnosis

The cause of infertility is an important factor affecting a woman's chance of success. If a clinic has little success in working with patients with endometriosis but is fantastic with ovulatory disorders, you want to know. In the sample report, there is less experience with unexplained infertility, but the doc has plenty of experience with ovulatory disorders (like PCOS). Patients with diminished ovarian reserve means they have high FSH or are tough responders to fertility medications.

Age

Your age dramatically influences your chances for success. Some clinics might have lower success rates because they specialize in more difficult cases, such as assisting older women become pregnant. As you consider clinics, look carefully at the statistics for your age group. Notice how the ages are divided in this report. As you can see, women older than forty-two are not included in the report. Women in this age group have virtually no chance of getting pregnant with IVF using their own eggs. However, older women can be included in the donor egg cycle since all ages are combined.

Types of Cycles

The cycles are usually divided into four sections: fresh and frozen nondonor eggs and fresh and frozen from donor eggs. Fresh eggs are those created and retrieved especially for this cycle. If there are leftover embryos, then they are frozen and saved for a FET (frozen embryo transfer). Pay attention to the statistics that closely resemble what you want to do.

The probability of having a baby with your own eggs starts to decline after age thirty-five and falls dramatically again after forty-one. About 15,000 couples a year use donor eggs to build their families, so it is critical to look at the types of procedures done (particularly nondonor eggs versus donor eggs) and their success rates for women at certain ages and with certain diagnoses. If you know or suspect you are going to need donor eggs, then focus specifically on those numbers. On the sample report, the rates are divided between fresh and frozen cycles, as well as donor and nondonor cycles.

Egg donation statistics are also a good sign of a successful clinic. Because most women who seek egg donation are older or have high FSH levels, by definition, selection cannot occur. If a program has low pregnancy rates for donor egg patients, it will most likely have low rates across all groups, alerting you of a problem. Frozen donor egg cycles on the sample report had a pregnancy rate of 37.5 percent, another sign of a good clinic.

Look for cancellation rates somewhere between 15 percent to 25 percent in women under forty. Cycles are canceled for many reasons: not enough follicles develop, embryos don't fertilize, or ovarian hyperstimulation or other problems occur. If the cancellation rate is zero, the clinic is lying. Much more than 25 percent and the clinic may not be adequately preparing patients. On this report, cancellation rates ranged from 13 percent to 22 percent.

PREGNANCY RATE

Look at the pregnancy rates for women under thirty-five. Although some women in this age group have high FSH levels or are poor responders, most should be able to become pregnant through IVF. As a result, pregnancy rates for younger women undergoing IVF should be significantly higher than for women over the age of thirty-five, indicating that the clinic treats a wide range of fertility issues across the age ranges. In the sample report, 41.3 percent of patients under thirty-five had a pregnancy, which is a respectable number.

Ignore small differences in pregnancy rates, say 44 percent versus 46 percent, because it isn't a statistically significant difference. Today, most good programs maintain a "take-home baby" rate of over 40 percent for women under thirty-five, and clinics you are considering should fall within that range. How low is too low? *Beware of programs with rates lower than 35 percent.* IVF success rates with frozen embryos should be similar to that of a fresh cycle as well.

Embryo Transfers

As you consider potential clinics, look carefully at the embryo transfer rate. Because of the hormones used to stimulate the production of lots of healthy eggs, twins, triplets, and other multiple pregnancies are more common in ARTs. The number of embryos transferred affects the multiple-birth rates; therefore, most clinics strive to transfer one or two embryos. *Be concerned with clinics which average more than 2.2 among women under the age of thirty-five.* On the sample report, 1.8 and 1.9 embryos on average were transferred.

Multiple Pregnancies

Despite the popular belief that multiples equal an instant family, there are difficulties, some of which are life-threatening, associated with multiples pregnancies. As one physician explains, "Right now in the NICU we have nineteen babies. Of these, only three are singleton births. We have two sets of triplets, and all the rest are twins. I can't tell you the number of times I've heard women express the desire for twins." Complications for Mom include pregnancy-induced hypertension, gestational diabetes, and placental problems, while babies are at risk for higher preterm birth rates and more negative health outcomes. Good clinics recognize these risks and do all they can to maintain low multiple-birth rates.

Overall, most clinics have multiple-birth rates of around 20 percent, with nearly all of these being twins. Be wary of any clinic reporting more than a handful of triplets or higher. The sample report indicates a twin rate of 29 percent and a triplet rate of 0 percent. Your main goal is to have a safe pregnancy and *one* healthy baby.

Current Clinic Services and Profile

This section summarizes what the clinic offers beyond traditional IVF, including donor eggs, donor embryos, and gestational carriers. It also mentions whether a clinic is able to freeze your embryos (cryopreservation), an important consideration if you think you might want to freeze any left-over embryos. SART membership and lab accreditation are also listed. Just because a clinic is not a member of SART or is not listed as having lab accreditation is not necessarily a deal breaker, but it is certainly an important question to ask when interviewing the clinic. Finally, the report also indicates if the clinic accepts single women. This piece of information can also be used as a proxy for their openness in treating gay men and lesbians. From our experience, those clinics that choose not to treat single women are less likely to support nontraditional relationships or lifestyles.

A Sample Report

Here is one clinic's annual report, given to the CDC. It is divided into sections tabulating overall treatment and diagnosis, and then subsections on fresh and frozen cycles for nondonor eggs and donor eggs.

I. ART Cycle Profile

TYPE OF ART	PROCEDURAL FACTORS	PATIENT DIAGNOSIS
IVF: 100 percent	With ICSI: 40 percent	Tubal factor: 9 percent
GIFT: 0 percent	Unstimulated: 0 percent	Ovulatory dysfunction: 19 percent
ZIFT: 0 percent	Used Gestational Carrier: 0 percent	Diminished ovarian reserve: 4 percent
Combination: 0 percent		Endometriosis: 4 percent
		Uterine factor: 0 percent
		Male factor: 4 percent
		Other factor: 3 percent
		Unknown factor: <1 percent
		Multiple factors: 25 percent
		Female factors only: 25 percent
		Female and male factors: 32 percent

II. Pregnancy Success Rates

FRESH EMBRYOS FROM NONDONOR EGGS

	AGE OF WOMAN			
	<35	35–37	38–40	41–42
Number of cycles	121	41	27	6
Percentage of cycles resulting in pregnancies	41.3	29.3	29.6	0/6

	AGE OF WOMAN			
	<35	**35–37**	**38–40**	**41–42**
Percentage of cycles resulting in live births	39.7	22.0	18.5	0/6
(Confidence Interval)	(30.0–49.0)	(10.6–37.6)	(6.3–38.1)	-
Percentage of retrievals resulting in live births	45.7	28.1	21.7	0/2
Percentage of transfers resulting in live births	50.5	33.3	23.8	-
Percentage of transfers resulting in live singleton births	35.8	18.5	23.8	-
Percentage of cancellations	12.2	22.0	14.8	4/6
Average number of embryos transferred	1.9	1.9	1.8	-
Percentage of pregnancies with twins	30.0	5/12	0/8	-
Percentage of pregnancies with triplets or more	0	0/12	0/8	-
Percentage of live births having multiple infants	29.2	4/9	0/5	-

FROZEN EMBRYOS FROM NONDONOR EGGS

	AGE OF WOMAN			
	<35	**35–37**	**38–40**	**41–42**
Number of transfers	23	6	7	0
Percentage of transfers resulting in live births	21.7	3/6	2/7	0
Average number of embryos transferred	1.8	1.5	2.0	-

DONOR EGGS

	ALL AGES COMBINED	
	FRESH EMBRYOS	**FROZEN EMBRYOS**
Number of transfers	5	24
Percentage of transfers resulting in live births	2.5	37.5
Average number of embryos transferred	1.4	1.9

III. Current Clinic Services and Profile

Donor egg?	Yes
Donor embryo?	Yes
Gestational carrier?	No
Cryopreservation?	Yes
SART Member?	Yes
Verified lab accreditation?	Yes
Single women?	Yes

Success by Any Other Name

If the clinic you are interested in boasts "success" rates of 50 percent, what does that mean? Do half of all women bring home a baby, or do they just get pregnant and then miscarry? You are interested in the actual take-home baby rate, but some success stats are confusing. Here are some other terms clinics use to describe their success rates.

- **Live birth rate per egg stimulation:** how many births occur in relation to the number of egg-stimulation procedures performed. It includes all live births as well as all procedures performed, including those that failed.
- **Live birth rate per embryo transfer:** this is the percentage of births from all embryo transfer procedures. It does not include those instances where the procedure did not succeed or was canceled.
- **Pregnancy rate per attempted egg stimulation:** the number of clinical pregnancies resulting from all egg-stimulation attempts. These clinical pregnancies include all those women with at least one positive pregnancy test even if the pregnancy ended in miscarriage.
- **Pregnancy rate per woman in program:** how many clinical pregnancies occurred per woman in the program—*not* how many procedures it took to get pregnant or if those women actually delivered a baby.
- **Pregnancy rate per attempted egg retrieval:** the number of clinical pregnancies resulting from all egg-retrieval attempts.

Again, pregnancy is counted, not babies. This also doesn't include failed cycles where no eggs were retrieved.

- **Pregnancy rate per embryo transfer:** how many pregnancies occurred in relation to the number of embryo-transfer procedures performed. This doesn't count babies or cycle attempts.

The Ugly Side of Statistics

Fertility clinics are for-profit companies that carefully select what information to release. No one looks over their collective shoulders to verify it is done accurately or even done at all. More than one fertility specialist we spoke to suggested it is commonly acknowledged that some success rates are fudged. Fertility clinics are in the business to make money, and they want your business. To do so, their stats need to look great.

How Fertility Clinics Create Good Statistics
(Adapted from the Genetics and IVF Institute at www.GIVF.com)

1. Classify difficult patients as research subjects.
2. Move challenging patients to donor egg services early.
3. Discourage embryo cryopreservation.
4. Attract better patients with a "refund package."
5. Enrich the patient population with the best patients (e.g., have low FSH cutoffs).
6. Use a waiting list where good patients go to the head of the line, and more challenging patients are either rejected or put on hold.
7. Encourage or require cancellation when follicle response is limited.
8. Encourage patients who are poor responders to exit the program.
9. Transfer larger numbers (usually well over two) of embryos to the uterus.

You won't know for sure if your clinic refused to take patients who weren't easy to "fix," nor will you know how reliable the numbers are. Learn to read between the lines. If it's too good to be true, be suspicious.

Dr. Joseph D. Schulman, founder of the Genetics and IVF Institute in Fairfax, Virginia, created the following table to suggest how IVF programs

> ## HOW PATIENT SELECTION WORKS
>
> A thirty-nine-year-old woman was turned away from a clinic due to age and told to return next year when she was forty. Why? Even though her personal odds of conception diminished slightly by waiting, her odds of success were still good. Since statistical reports lump all women over forty into one group, her likely success would do more good for the clinic's success rate as a forty-year-old than as a thirty-nine-year-old.

that are identical in ability can look very different when one of the centers "cherry-picks" its clients.

In Dr. Schulman's example, "Dr. Lookgood" looks about twice as good in a number of his statistics. Yet "Dr. Helpall" treats patients according to a philosophy typical of medicine in most other fields: take patients in the order they come to you, help those who have a chance of being helped, do your best for each individual patient, and let the population statistics fall where they may. It won't be initially obvious whether you are seeing Dr. Lookgood or Dr. Helpall unless you do your homework and find out more about your clinic's statistics and what factors are driving these numbers.

WHO IS REALLY LOOKING OUT FOR YOUR BEST INTERESTS? It's easy to be impressed by seemingly good-looking success rates. After all, all you really want is a baby to take home. First, let's look at the final "pregnancy rate" stats of two very different doctors, Dr. Lookgood and Dr. Helpall.

	DR. LOOKGOOD	DR. HELPALL
Percentage of pregnancies per embryo transfer	42	21
Percentage of pregnancies per egg retrieval	40	19
Percentage of pregnancies per IVF cycle	28	18
Percentage of births per embryo transfer	33	15

	DR. LOOKGOOD	DR. HELPALL
Percentage of births per egg retrieval	31	13
Percentage of births per IVF cycle	22	13

You are probably thinking, "Wow! I'm going with Dr. Lookgood. She is twice as good as Dr. Helpall." Unfortunately, as with much in life, things are not always what they seem. Let's look at these statistics a little more closely and evaluate all that goes into influencing these numbers. (We have added our own commentary in italics to Dr. Schulman's original example so you can get a clearer understanding of exactly what is going on here.)

	DR. LOOKGOOD	DR. HELPALL
Total number of patients who called the clinic for an appointment	100	100
Number of patients who were seen by the doctor	80 *Twenty percent were told by the receptionist that they were "not good candidates for this program" before they could even schedule their first appointment.*	96 *Nearly all the patients who called the clinic were encouraged to come in for an initial appointment with the doctor.*
Number of patients accepted into the program	60 *Another 25 percent were told there were "not good candidates for this program" after their first appointment.*	94 *Nearly all the patients who were seen by the doctor were encouraged to participate in the program.*
Number of patients whose cycles promptly started	50 *For 17 percent, the doctor did not start their cycle at all because she did not think the situation was "ideal" so she wanted to stop and try again at another time.*	94 *Nearly all the patients were able to start their cycles on time.*

	DR. LOOKGOOD	DR. HELPALL
Number of patients whose cycles were NOT canceled	35 *Another 30 percent of cycles were canceled after the cycle was started probably because the doctor thought there were too few eggs produced to proceed.*	90 *In nearly all the cases, the doctor encouraged the cycle once the patient had started the fertility medications no matter how many eggs developed. After all, technically speaking, you only need one good egg.*
Number of patients who had embryos transferred	33 *Two patients did not have any embryos transferred because the doctor thought none were "good enough" to transfer.*	80 *Unfortunately, ten patients clearly had no embryos survive. For the other 89 percent, the doctor transferred the best-looking embryos that had made it that far in hopes that something would work.*
Number of patients who had four or more embryos transferred	31 *Nearly all the patients had four or more embryos transferred, which significantly increases the rates of multiple births and further complications for both mother and babies.*	10 *In only a few extenuating circumstances (for example, several failed IVF cycles), the doctor agreed to transfer back more than four embryos. This was done only after careful consideration and communication with the patients about the risks involved.*
Number of patients who became pregnant	14 *Due to the high number of embryos transferred, many of these pregnancies were multiples.*	17 *Seventeen patients became pregnant, with only one being a twin pregnancy.*
Number of patients who gave birth.	11 *Due to premature births, most of the multiples endured long NICU stays and subsequent long-term problems.*	12 *Only the twin pregnancy experienced complications.*

In the end, the actual take-home baby numbers for both doctors are almost identical. However, Dr. Helpall truly wants to help all his patients have a baby despite their unique situation or individual chance of success. On the other hand, Dr. Lookgood stacks her numbers by selecting only those patients she feels have the greatest chance for success and taking greater risks that might harm the patient.

HOW TO ASSESS YOUR CLINIC'S STATISTICS

- Ask exactly how success rates are calculated and evaluate all claims carefully.
- Some clinics cite only national statistics when discussing success rates. Be wary of claims not based on your clinic's own numbers.
- Pay attention to success rates for people who fit your particular patient profile, particularly your age and cause of infertility.
- Consider cost. "Expensive" does not necessarily equate with "best quality."

"Look at success rates, but as a potential patient and consumer, consider all the important factors and influences when choosing whom to trust with your infertility care," explains Dr. Schulman. "What is most important is the experience and expertise of the IVF team, the experiences of your fellow patients, the overall reputation of the program, and your own intuitive response to the physicians and other professionals with whom you come into contact."

> *"Clinics are so variable in who they accept, the statistics are almost meaningless. I was turned away from four clinics near me because of weight, yet got pregnant from my very first IVF—with no other treatment whatsoever—at the one in my home state . . . just think, I could have been one of those positive stats those clinics like to use. Oh well, their loss—my very happy gain!"*
>
> —SUSAN

Old data is another problem with statistics. While these data are compiled every year, there is a lag time between when the reports are submitted and when they become available to the public. Consequently, the statistics are already up to two or three years old by the time you read them. During this time, clinics could have changed in terms of protocols, staffing, laboratory techniques, and overall quality.

You can request more recent statistical reports directly from each fertility clinic that you are considering. Also, ask for reports from previous years to look for trends in the data over time. Year-to-year data can reveal information on the quality, stability, and experience of the program. Ask for the most recent CDC statistics for your age based on delivery rate per embryo transfer.

WILL IT WORK FOR ME?

How will you know if you will be successful? Because everyone's situation is different, there is no way to predict how successful your cycle will be. Factors that make it more likely to be successful include: being a healthy non-smoker, previous pregnancy with IVF, egg donor, or younger age.

AVERAGE IVF SUCCESS RATES*

35–39: 33 percent
40–42: 15 percent
Over 42: 5 percent

*Source: WebMD at www.webmd.com

You have poorer chances of success if you are older and using your own eggs, have a history of recurrent miscarriage, both male and female factor infertility, multiple previously unsuccessful IVF attempts, uterine abnormality (DES exposure, fibroids), or ovarian dysfunction (high FSH level). But there is no formula that we can use to tell you whether or not this will work. Our best advice: be optimistic, yet realistic.

The More the Merrier?: Different Types of Clinics

Fertility clinics come in all sizes and with all kinds of reputations. There is no absolute right or wrong as to which type of clinic is best. They all have their pros and cons. Once you have reviewed statistical data on clinics you are interested in, you may want to look more closely at the type of clinic you are considering.

The Sole Practitioner

Some fertility specialists practice alone. These docs might be able to provide you with more personalized attention and the luxury of really getting to know you and your unique situation. Experiences vary, but many doctors in solo practices often get great reviews for staying connected to their patients via emails and are even known to give out their cell phone numbers. No promises, but you will probably have greater access to your doctor than you would in a larger practice. The biggest advantage is that individual doctors who do not operate within an institutionalized system are much more willing and able to negotiate prices.

These smaller clinics also have fewer resources than much larger practices. In terms of your wallet, you might have to pay additional costs (and deal with additional bills from various companies or practices) if they contract out their lab work, testing, embryology, or coverage for when they aren't available. You might be more restricted as to when you can make appointments or schedule procedures if you're dependent on one doctor.

Large, Full-Service Practices

Larger infertility clinics have anywhere from two to ten fertility specialists and a host of additional staff. Typically, they will offer more in-house services and laboratories. They may be open more hours, offer various office locations for greater convenience and accessibility to services. The best benefit is your doctor will have a number of colleagues with equally strong credentials for possible consultations and backup if he or she is unavailable.

The drawback? With several specialists in the practice, you might not see the same physician at each visit, and your primary fertility specialist might not be available to answer your questions directly. Don't expect personal calls or emails from your doc. Instead, your message will probably be handed off to nurses and medical assistants who will call when they can. Multiple offices, extra staff, expensive décor, and slick marketing aren't free. Although the costs are spread across more patients, you are paying for it. Know that if you choose a larger clinic, fees might be higher to cover the overhead, and you might get lost in the shuffle of their many patients.

Fertility Networks

Many clinics throughout the United States have banded together to form fertility networks. These networks, which can be found throughout the country, allow clinics to pool their resources to offer more coordinated care. While networks typically benefit physicians more than patients, there are some advantages to clinics that are part of a network. There are two main national fertility networks currently available: Advanced Reproductive Care (or ARC) and IntegraMed.

These companies offer the most help to patients when it comes to financing their fertility treatment. They offer services ranging from package pricing, refund guarantees, risk sharing, and monthly payment programs. While you may get more help financing the treatment, clinics in these networks are less likely to negotiate the price of their services. If you have a hard time coming up with traditional financing or you need assistance with developing a realistic payment plan, working with an organization like ARC or IntegraMed is a good choice. To find out more information, contact them directly or ask your fertility clinic if they participate in one of these networks.

- Advanced Reproductive Care (ARC): www.arcfertility.com
- IntegraMed: www.integramed.com

An alternative model, often referred to as the McDonald's of the infertility industry, involves a few fertility specialists who have utilized their entrepreneurial skills to develop national chains of fertility clinics with locations across the country. Because of sheer patient volume, these clinics are able to offer several perks for their patients, including twenty-four-hour phone access to nurses, an innovative and extensive website, electronic recordkeeping, free initial consultations, and money-back guarantees. Critics argue that these types of clinics are more interested in quantity of patients than the quality of care.

Hospital-Based Clinics

Large community hospitals are beginning to share space with independent laboratories, outpatient surgery centers, and other specialty health groups, including fertility clinics. Doctors often join together and may look for locations that are associated with an established hospital. If people are used to going to the hospital and affiliated medical offices for other types of care, they might be more willing to seek out infertility treatments there as well. By sharing resources with the hospital and other doctors, costs are reduced, which may result in lower prices for patients but not always. Hospital-based clinics may also make it more difficult to coordinate care due to the increased bureaucracy and red tape, especially with regard to scheduling, insurance, and billing.

Patients are also able to utilize other resources located on the hospital campus, such as nearby laboratories, radiologists, and surgical centers, in addition to broader reproductive services, obstetrical care, and, eventually, pediatricians. However, just because they are located beside each other doesn't mean the fertility clinic has the same reputation as the hospital, or vice versa. Assess the clinic independently, on its own merits.

University-Based Clinics

Technically, university-based clinics are considered nonprofit, but don't let the name fool you. Their prices are consistent with other types of clinics in the same area. On the bright side, some university-based clinics are involved with federally funded research or they network with other clinics, which could give you a break in treatment costs or the opportunity to try more cutting-edge treatments.

Because university-based clinics are teaching institutions, prepare to have medical students and residents in your exam room. If your clinic participates in educating future fertility specialists, your doctor might even allow them to do the exam or treatment. Another downside is that the fertility center may share a waiting room with general ob-gyn patients, which means you might be surrounded by pregnant women.

While university-based clinics attract some of the best and brightest names in reproductive medicine and research, many clinics find themselves in jeopardy as physicians leave to pursue more lucrative private practices. Recently, a major midwestern university closed its fertility clinic due to cost cutting and left three thousand patients suddenly scrambling to find care elsewhere. Don't assume that because a clinic is associated with a prestigious university, it provides exceptional care. It may be no better than any other clinic, plus you will be subjected to a lot more red tape. Look at a university-based fertility clinic with the same scrutiny as you would any other.

First Impressions

"From the moment of our first meeting, I felt distinctly as if I was the second most important person in the room, next to himself. I had done my fair share of research ahead of time, but when sitting across from our doctor, I suddenly felt very inadequate. Not only did he speak incredibly fast, rattling off acronyms I had never heard, but he also refused to make eye contact with us. With promises of pregnancy flowing from his mouth, we wrongly decided if the end result was the family we had dreamed, we could easily deal with our doctor's ego."

—Jenna

Call clinics you're interested in and ask for additional information. Begin to assess them during this first phone call. It's never too early to ask the tough financial questions so you can better gauge what you are getting yourself into.

First impressions are important: don't ever underestimate your gut feelings. For example, how were you greeted: behind a glass partition with no eye contact or by someone who was happy you walked in the door? After all, this commitment is going to last several months to several years and will involve an investment of thousands of dollars out of your pocket. Find a clinic you trust to take good care of you physically, emotionally, and financially.

Initial Considerations
- Was the staff courteous and happy to talk to you?
- Did the staff seem willing to answer your questions and interested in you personally?
- What is the wait time for a first appointment?
- How accessible will the staff be to you in terms of appointment times and call-backs? (Fertility clinics should be available to you 24/7, especially since women don't ovulate only between 9 a.m. and 5 p.m. Monday through Friday.)

- Does the practice have any restrictions on who is seen (and many do) in terms of age, marital status, sexual orientation, or certain health conditions?

Most fertility clinics have websites which should be checked out as well. Read all the information they provide, including the practice philosophy, physician and staff profiles, and treatment descriptions. The most helpful sites offer information on pricing, financing, and insurance companies with whom they have relationships.

Often, fertility clinics will offer free informational events on infertility-related topics. Keep tabs on any clinic within a reasonable travel distance from you. Sign up for email newsletters or other updates. Whenever events are offered, try to attend. Besides getting to meet the physician or other staff, you might learn something new.

The Bottom Line

Treating infertility is complex, and the decision about where to go for treatment can be even more complex. Comfort with the clinic and staff, cost, and success rates are all key factors in making your decision. By making the first step an informed one, you can save far more than money alone.

Five Things You Can Do Right Now
1. Ask medical professionals and friends for referrals.
2. Review CDC and SART statistics for clinics that interest you.
3. Gather information online from blogs, bulletin boards, and clinic websites.
4. Narrow down your clinic choices to the top five.
5. Start making calls to gather more specific information.

CHAPTER 4

You Are Not Alone:
Create a Team That Works for You

"Yesterday Tim and I had our IVF classes. We started the day with a two-hour class with the embryologist and four other couples. We were given the details about her job, good eggs, bad eggs, ICSI, embryo quality, and an assortment of extras that could be added on in the lab, depending upon how things look.

"After the meeting with the embryologist, Tim and I met with the office manager to discuss the money. My insurance covers some parts of the cycle, such as blood work and ultrasounds, but we will still be paying at least $9,250 out of pocket for the procedure.

"Next, we met with the fertility specialist for a quick review of our plan, then we saw the nurse practitioner. She gave us a rough outline of our protocol and explained all of the medications, how they would be administered, and what their risks and side effects were. My mind is spinning knowing that I will have to keep up with a grand total of eleven prescription meds over the coming weeks. I barely remember to take my stupid prenatal vitamins every day.

"After lunch, we came back, and Tim had to endure another semen analysis (puh-lease!), and then we spent the afternoon in the IVF injection class taught by some of the nurses. Although we already knew that five of the meds must be injected, we were still horrified by the sight of the progesterone needle. I knew it was an inch and a half long, but actually seeing it, live and in person, was a little intimidating.

"We left the office late afternoon, feeling a little overwhelmed. We are excited and nervous and hopeful, but it's so weird to know twelve different people are going to be involved in making our baby. I don't even remember all their names."

—KIM

Because infertility is a multibillion-dollar business, a lot of people are interested in your infertility for a variety of reasons. Most genuinely care and want to help you achieve your dream of having a baby. We hate to admit it, but with thousands of dollars at stake, others may be taking advantage of your situation. How do you know who is who? And with infertility treatment being so expensive, you can't afford to waste money on anyone or anything unproductive.

In this chapter, we will introduce you to all the possible people who may be involved with your overall fertility plan. We will provide you with tips about how to best spend your money and allocate other equally scarce resources, such as time and energy. Creating a good team and maintaining control over your game plan from the beginning not only protects your money but also saves time, reduces the emotional burden, and increases the likelihood of bringing a new child into your family.

First Things First: Your Clinic Staff

Once you have narrowed down your list of potential clinics, you need to carefully assess the doctors and his or her staff. Dr. Zev Rosenwaks, director of the Center for Reproductive Medicine and Infertility at New York Weill Cornell, explains, "I've never felt the facility where the doctor practices makes a difference. It's a doctor and program that make a difference. It's the doctors' backgrounds, where they were trained, their experience, the experience of their team. So I think whether it's private or university is less important than looking at the individuals involved and the type of program."

Some fertility specialists will insist infertility care is dependent on the high-tech equipment. "We all have the same tools," explains Dr. James Donahue of Family Beginnings in Indianapolis. "We all have a microscope—granted, it's a really good one, but there are only two main brands. And we have an incubator. Again, there isn't a lot of leeway in cost on these. You spend about $300,000 outfitting your clinic, but it's a fixed cost."

The other fixed expense is staffing. Besides the physician, an average IVF center has at least seven additional staff to support the fertility specialist: an embryologist, billing coordinator, receptionist, office manager, two nurses, and a mental health specialist. Salaries can depend on the location of the clinic and the experience and expertise of the staff. That doesn't include the cost of public relations and marketing, or attorney costs and professional membership fees.

What's left? The profit. "Some clinics charge $8,000 [per IVF cycle] because they can and that's what the market will bear. They are willing to accept that fewer patients have access to care," says Dr. Donahue. But he does things a little differently. "I can charge $4,000 and still make money. I live well. I drive a BMW. But I also treat people who would never be able to afford the other fertility center across town."

The Fertility Specialist

Becoming a fertility specialist requires four years of college followed by four years of medical school, a four-year residency in obstetrics and gynecology, and then a three-year fellowship in reproductive endocrinology and infertility. Only fertility specialists who are board certified (in other words, they passed an exam assessing their knowledge about reproductive endocrinology and infertility) can use the title reproductive endocrinologist, or RE. It's important to ask because not all fertility specialists are board certified in reproductive endocrinology and infertility. Also, a fertility specialist should be up on the latest research, regularly reading scientific journals and attending professional meetings.

IMPORTANCE OF BOARD CERTIFICATION

In addition to completing years of schooling, fulfilling residency requirements, and passing the exams required to practice medicine in your state, your board-certified specialist participates in an ongoing process of continuing education to keep current with the latest advances in medical science and technology in his or her specialty as well as the best practices in patient safety, quality health care, and creating a responsive patient-focused environment. To maintain board certification, your physician participates in an extensive process that involves completing accredited education and specialty training and periodic oral and written exams to demonstrate competency. To find out if your physician is board certified, contact the American Board of Medical Specialties at www.abms.org or 1-866-ASK-ABMS.

In terms of salaries, fertility specialists are well paid. They are typically consistent with other highly specialized physicians such as cardiothoracic, plastic, and orthopedic surgeons. A fertility specialist can expect to start at $250,000 right out of school, and average along the lines of $375,000 a year after a few years of experience. It is not unheard of for fertility specialist salaries to top the million-dollar mark, especially if they own their own clinics. In contrast, a family physician's salary ranges from $100,000 to $200,000.

There is no doubt that fertility specialists spent a lot of time and effort to get where they are, and their expertise doesn't come cheap. The bottom line is the reason your clinic charges so much money may have more to do with your physician's wallet than with the latest piece of high-tech equipment. Just because some doctors have stellar creds and drive fancy cars doesn't mean they provide top-notch services. As with service providers across the board, from hairstylists to lawyers, skill levels vary. Ask the tough questions, expect answers, and don't fall for the old line, "Trust me, I'm the doctor."

Reproductive Urologist

A reproductive urologist is a medical doctor with additional training in treating urinary tract and male reproductive disorders. Fertility clinics must have access to a urologist who specializes in diagnosing and treating male factor problems. While it is not critical that the urologist be officially on staff, the urologist must work closely with the clinic to ensure that treatment of the couple is a coordinated effort.

Embryologist and Andrologist

Most of us don't think about the people hidden back in the lab, but an embryologist can be the deciding factor in whether or not you get pregnant using ARTs. The embryologist is ultimately responsible for preparing the sperm, fertilizing the eggs, growing the embryos, caring for them until they are ready to be transferred, and carefully freezing any extras. It requires a tremendous amount of concentration, dedication, and skill. One slipup, and your chances are gone, no matter how good your fertility specialist. Unlike fertility specialists, who must have a medical degree to practice, an embryologist can have a bachelor's degree, master's degree, or doctorate in clinical embryology. Not surprisingly, salaries rise significantly with additional education and experience.

Ask about the number of laboratory procedures your embryologist typically does in a year. Most experienced embryologists will be doing well more than twenty complete ART cycles per year. They should also be well versed in successfully freezing and thawing embryos with a survival rate of more than 50 percent. An outstanding embryologist will also be actively attending conferences, participating in research, and publishing the results of this research along with presenting it to his or her peers. When you are looking at clinics, ask for credentials and to speak with the embryologist one-on-one.

Fertility clinics also utilize an andrologist. Andrologists are similar to embryologists in that they are trained laboratory specialists. The andrologist's focus is hormonal issues and sperm quality related to male-factor infertility. These professionals develop and direct procedures for handling sperm, where they work closely with the embryologist to prepare sperm up to the point of fertilization.

Quick Tip!
You can verify each clinic's lab accreditation on the CDC and SART clinic ART reports.

Laboratory certification is another important factor. The lab should be in good standing with any licensing or accreditation boards, such as the Commission on Laboratory Accreditation or the College of American Pathologists. Most important, every fertility clinic should have a certified high-complexity lab director (HCLD). Be skeptical of any clinic that does not employ one or depends solely on an "off-site" HCLD.

NURSE PRACTITIONERS AND PHYSICIAN'S ASSISTANTS

Because all fertility specialists are busy, some are beginning to employ what they call midlevel providers or physician extenders. This is a growing trend in medicine, and fertility clinics are no exception. Nurse practitioners and physician's assistants are able to do routine tasks, such as performing exams, diagnosing problems, ordering and interpreting tests, and in some cases even prescribing medications—all under the direct guidance of the fertility specialist. This allows physicians more time to concentrate on higher-level tasks only a trained physician can do, such as the actual infertility treatments.

In terms of the fertility clinic, physician extenders are a huge benefit. They are able to provide similar services as a physician while cutting some costs in the payroll department. However, know that this savings is usually not passed along to patients. Although many patients enjoy working with nurse practitioners and physician's assistants, you still have the right to see your physician at any time. Since you are spending a lot of money here, be wary if you are spending the majority of your time and money seeing a physician extender instead of your fertility specialist.

Other Medical Professionals

Fertility clinics are full of medical professionals ready to help you get that baby. These men and women (not surprisingly, many women are drawn to this type of job) will be your initial resource for getting answers and information.

Ask if your clinic is one of the few that has a **patient advocate,** or initial contact person, to help you get started with your treatment plan. A patient advocate is a valuable resource and can help you navigate through all aspects of your fertility care as well as act as an intermediary between you and the rest of the clinic staff.

A **nurse** or medical assistant in a fertility office provides patient education and emotional support, manages care, monitors and tracks patients, maintains communication between physicians and patients, and receives and communicates test results. Your nursing staff will be the gatekeepers, allowing you access to your doctor and additional information. When you go to a fertility clinic, ask the nursing staff what drew them to this specialization, how long they have worked in this field, and if they enjoy their job. You should find their answers comforting and encouraging, particularly since you will spend more time with them than with the physician. Fertility nurses should possess superior communication skills. Do not underestimate their importance in your care.

Because fertility specialists address genetic concerns with their patients, a **genetic counselor** might also be on staff. A master's-level genetic counselor can provide you with more specific information regarding any genetic concerns you have or testing that has been done. This is especially important if you have suffered multiple miscarriages or have a family history of genetic disorders.

Some fertility clinics employ a **pharmacist** to manage all of the fertility-related prescriptions. This prevents possible miscommunication between the prescribing physician and the pharmacy. They can ensure you are getting exactly what they are prescribing and your questions are answered accurately about what, when, and how you take your meds.

AVERAGE ANNUAL SALARIES OF FERTILITY CLINICAL STAFF

Reproductive Endocrinologist or Fertility Specialist: $350,000 to $1,000,000
Urologist: $200,000+
Pharmacist: $100,000
Embryologist: $60,000 to $70,000
Nurse Practitioner or Physician's Assistant: $60,000 to $70,000
Andrologist: $50,000
Nurse Egg Donor Coordinator: $50,000
Genetic Counselor: $50,000
Nurse: $40,000
Medical Assistant: $30,000

NONCLINICAL STAFF

In addition to the medical staff, fertility clinics also count on a number of nonclinical staff to keep things running. This includes receptionists, office or practice administrators, financial counselors (who deal with insurance and billing), and maybe even a marketing and/or public relations staff to attract more patients. The larger the clinic, the more nonmedical staff it usually employs. Even if this allows the clinic to provide good customer service, somebody has to pay for them. Part of your bill pays their paychecks. In addition, the more staff in a clinic, the more people there will be between you and your doctor. In other words, it may be more difficult to speak directly with your doctor.

You will be interacting with these staff members during the administrative parts of your treatment—setting up appointments, dealing with bills, checking on test results, and trying to get in touch with your doctor or nurse. We've all been there, and dealing with administration and bureaucracy can be time-consuming and extremely frustrating, especially when you aren't getting the results you want. These feelings of frustration are further magnified when you are stressed out, which you always are when trying to have a baby! Mood swings (a side effect of many fertility drugs) don't help either.

> *"Having to ask patients for their payments is the worst part of my job. I hate seeing the looks in people's eyes when I have to tell them I need a check for $15,000 before they can even schedule their next appointment. Sometimes they cry. Other times I know they are cursing me under their breaths. I wish they could understand this is painful for me as well."*
> —Dawn, fertility clinic financial coordinator

If a staff member gives you bad news, don't shoot the messenger. They don't make the rules. Like the rest of us working stiffs, they are trying to do their job the best they can, often under difficult circumstances. If you get on their bad side, they will not be motivated to help you get what you want. Try to be patient, pleasant, and understanding. You get more results (and faster too!) if you play nice. If you have a real complaint or concern, take it to the big brass—the fertility specialist. The fertility specialist is the only one with any power to make a change.

Third-Party Reproduction

If you decide to pursue any type of third-party reproduction (sperm donor, egg donor, embryo donor, and/or surrogate/gestational carrier), you will need more than doctors and nurses. Fertility clinics rarely work with sperm donors directly, so if you need donor sperm, you will need to contact an independent sperm donor agency. Some clinics have established relationships with certain sperm donor programs and will encourage you (or, in rare cases, require you) to work with them. Likewise, while a handful of clinics are involved with assisting patients in finding a surrogate or gestational carrier, this is not the norm. If you need a surrogate or gestational carrier, you are pretty much on your own to find an agency to assist you.

On the other hand, you have several options for finding an egg donor. Nearly all fertility clinics offer egg donation. Sometimes fertility clinics hire more specialized medical staff to manage their egg donor program. Nurses often serve as coordinators of clinic-run egg donor programs and are responsible for recruiting, screening, and matching you with potential egg donors. By using this type of egg donor program, you have all the benefits of one-stop shopping and more seamless coordination of the egg donation process from start to finish. Because clinics have a hard time recruiting donors, you will have fewer choices and longer wait times. In order to expedite the selection process, the donor coordinator will narrow down your options and may present you with only the ones she thinks best match the needs of your family. This can include height and weight, hair and eye color, complexion, education, interests, ethnicity, and family background. She will allow you to look only at these preselected files in order to make your choice.

If you decide to utilize an independent agency, this will provide you with more donor choices. However, you will have to pay the additional administration fees that support these agencies. Also, there are no guidelines or quality assurances as to third-party reproduction agencies, and some are better than others. A few are founded and administered by health care professionals who have experience in this area. Others are run by former patients or other interested people with little or no professional expertise.

Depending on your needs and desires, there are no easy answers. Be an informed consumer. Don't be fooled by good-looking marketing materials or fall for empty promises. Not everyone is looking out for your best interests. Critically evaluate a company's credentials, experience, track records, references, and how it treats its donors. Search online forums for any red flags and always ask to speak with previous clients. Above all, choose a professional, experienced, well-managed, and ethical agency.

YOUR MENTAL HEALTH

Infertility is not only physically arduous, it is also emotionally difficult. Infertility hits us at our very core and challenges us in ways we never imagined. Throughout the infertility journey, we are forced to make decisions affecting us and our families now and into the future. It's normal to feel that we cannot walk this road alone. Fortunately, there are many resources out there to help through these difficult times.

MENTAL HEALTH CLINICIANS

Good mental health is a key component of a successful infertility experience. In general, be suspicious of any clinic that does not take your mental health concerns seriously. The medical professionals should not only recognize your mental health needs, but they should also provide you with resources to seek appropriate mental health care. Because of the tremendous emotional toll that infertility will take on you, this is no place to cut expenses.

Clinics recognize this and may have a mental health clinician on staff to meet with patients who are participating in any type of assisted reproductive technology, including IVF, egg donation, and surrogacy as well as throughout the treatment process. In these cases, the cost of meeting with a mental health professional should be included in the overall cost of your treatment, although it is always smart to ask.

If a clinic does not have a mental health clinician on staff or requires you to undergo an initial evaluation, it should be able to provide you with a list of local clinicians who routinely work with infertility patients. If the clinic provides you with a list, call around and inquire about pricing. How many times will you be required to meet? What are the costs—is it hourly or a fixed price? The costs will typically be in the $100 to $200 per appointment range, but you might luck out and find one on the lower end. Mental health professionals can include social workers, family therapists, clinical psychologists, trained counselors, and psychiatrists. Obviously, a practitioner's specific education, credentials, and experience will be reflected in their fees. The American Society for Reproductive Medicine (ASRM) offers a list of mental health professionals who specialize in infertility and other family-building issues (www.asrm.org).

SUPPORT GROUPS

Instead of meeting with a counselor one-on-one for ongoing support, you can opt to participate in support groups. Most infertility-related support groups consist of about five to fifteen people who gather regularly (once a week to once a month) to discuss and provide each other with support about some aspect of infertility. Some groups are very general discussions about infertility, while others are more specific and address topics like IVF, egg donation, or surrogacy. Groups can be women only, men only, or for couples. They can be led by trained professionals or by peers. They can be completely free or up to $50 a meeting. Check with your fertility clinic, your mental health professional, your local religious organization, or an infertility patient organization for more information about support groups. Find a support group in which you feel comfortable sharing your experiences and concerns.

COMPLEMENTARY AND ALTERNATIVE MEDICINE

Some infertility experts highlight the importance of relaxation and well-being in the overall success of infertility treatments. A few clinics even employ on-site acupuncturists or massage therapists. Other clinics develop relationships with certain complementary care professionals to whom they regularly refer patients.

For an acupuncturist, visits typically cost $75 to $100 per session and require multiple sessions over several weeks or months. Since acupuncture is not just a one-shot deal, this can easily add up to several thousands of dollars above your regular treatment costs. Likewise, a massage session costs at least $80 per one-hour session.

Dr. Alice Domar, founder of the Domar Center for Mind/Body Health and author of *Conquering Infertility: Dr. Alice Domar's Mind/Body Guide to Enhancing Fertility and Coping with Infertility*, suggests that utilizing certain mind-body techniques can provide a greater sense of well-being and help you be in a better place mentally and emotionally to deal with the stress of treatments. Many people strongly believe in the effects of such treatment approaches, whether used in place of or alongside more conventional medical treatments. If you choose this route, carefully select your practitioner and confirm she is licensed, experienced, and has a solid reputation, especially within the fertility field.

If you aren't able to seek complementary care due to financial constraints, you can achieve similar benefits through other lower-cost, stress-reducing techniques, such as tai chi, meditation, or yoga. You can join a group at your local gym, place of worship, or community center, or do it on your own using videos, tapes, or books.

Additional Professional Help

Since infertility is a complicated process, we need a little extra assistance in navigating through all the complexities. This requires professionals knowledgeable about the infertility industry. How do you find these people? Let's look at a few key areas:

LAWYERS

For standard infertility procedures, such as IUI and IVF, you don't need to hire an attorney. Although you will be required to sign a number of consent forms before your treatments start, these forms are standard and easy to understand. These consent forms are similar to what you would sign if you were undergoing any type of medical procedure, such as outpatient surgery. They contain information aimed at protecting you and the clinic (but mostly the clinic) from any complications in the event something goes wrong during or after the procedure.

Typical Consent Forms Include

- General consent (for both partners to give voluntary consent to the procedure that you understand the purpose of the procedure and any associated risks);
- Sedation consent (gives permission to give sedation or anesthesia);
- Cryopreservation of embryos (gives permission to freeze any remaining embryos and includes instructions about what will happen to the embryos after the treatments are completed);
- HIV consent (gives permission for HIV testing for both partners);
- Specific procedural request and authorization forms (describes procedure and any associated risks and gives permission for the clinic to perform various procedures such as IUI, egg retrieval, ICSI, fertilization, PGD, and embryo transfer).

For your own protection, read over everything very carefully. You can ask to take these forms home with you and take more time to carefully review them. If you have any questions or concerns, bring these up to the clinic staff immediately. Never sign anything you do not understand.

If you are going for *any type* of third-party reproduction involving some combination of sperm donors, egg donors, embryo donors, or surrogates/gestational carriers, hiring an attorney makes good financial sense. To protect against any unexpected complications or confusion after the baby is born regarding parental roles and responsibilities, you will need an attorney to draw up contracts specifying expectations and agreements. A little more money now can save you a lot later if problems arise.

THIRD-PARTY AGREEMENTS OR CONTRACTS SHOULD INCLUDE

- Donor gives up all rights to the genetic material (sperm, eggs, or embryos) and any children conceived from them.

- Donors have no right to custody or visitation and cannot be sued for child support.

- Intended parents will be financially responsible for the entire donation process, including counseling, medical costs, and prescription costs.

- If the donor is paid, the specific amount should be specified along with when the payment will be provided.

Also, attorneys who specialize in family building can help you connect with a donor or surrogate/gestational carrier directly. They often have large networks of professional colleagues who can help facilitate the process of locating a donor or surrogate/gestational carrier, screening her, and preparing her for the process. If you are considering this path, it's always good to ask. Many families are surprised how easy it is to locate a donor or gestational carrier through their attorney's office. A major advantage of this is cutting out the middleman (otherwise known as the third-party agency), further cutting costs.

How do you find an attorney? First, hire a law firm or individual attorney who specializes in infertility law. While it is a growing specialty area, most states have only a handful of attorneys with experience in infertility law. Because state laws vary, you want to hire an attorney familiar with and licensed to practice in your state. You can get suggestions from your local fertility clinic, infertility organizations, or the state bar association. Most of these attorneys also specialize in all aspects of family building, including adoption.

How much will it cost to hire an attorney? Before you meet with an attorney, always ask about fees. More specifically, it is also a good idea to have your lawyer give you a written estimate of anticipated costs. Different attorneys use different pay structures. Most attorneys charge by the hour. Not all attorneys charge the same hourly rate, so ask what their rate is and those of their support staff such as paralegals or on-staff experts. The hourly rates of attorneys vary widely depending on their expertise and level of experience. Even within a single law firm, hourly rates differ, with more experienced attorneys charging more per hour than more junior attorneys. On the other hand, some attorneys offer fixed fees for a set service, such as drawing up a contract between donor and recipient in third-party reproduction. Regardless of the fee structure, expect to pay a minimum of $2,000 in legal costs.

The amount you pay for a lawyer's services are the fee plus costs and expenses for your case. You should agree with your lawyer what costs are included in the fee before hiring. You may be able to negotiate the amount in advance for some of the costs.

HOW CAN YOU KEEP LEGAL COSTS DOWN?

- Be up front and honest with your attorney.

- Bring copies of all relevant documents with you to your meetings.

- Focus on business and get straight to the point.

- Write your questions down in advance and keep them brief.

FINANCIAL PLANNER

You do not need to hire a financial planner specifically to help you with this process. With a little bit of homework, you can easily gather all of this information on your own. Read financial books, scour the internet, or join a local club that deals with financial planning. Your bank or financial institution should also be able to provide you with free advice. All of this is much cheaper than forking over your cash to a financial planner.

If you already have a financial planner, discuss your overall family-building plans with her so she can incorporate these plans into your existing financial arrangements. If you decide you need objective third-party financial advice, find someone who is credentialed and experienced. Understand their fee structure and exactly what you will be getting for your money. A good planner should look at the big picture, taking into consideration investing, tax, and insurance issues and how it all relates to your overall family-building plans.

Most large fertility clinics have some sort of financial person on staff. Take advantage of this service (especially since you are already paying for it as part of your treatment costs). Make an appointment and see what she has to say. Ask for a written estimate of all itemized costs associated with your individual treatment plan. Perhaps she can give you a few new ideas or tips about creative financing solutions. Still, know that this person is being paid by the clinic and has the clinic's best interest in mind, so any information provided will be biased.

INFERTILITY CONSULTANTS AND COACHES

While certainly not the most cost-effective investment, this may be a reasonable option for someone who has more money than time. If you feel overwhelmed, aren't willing to scour insurance papers with a fine-tooth comb, and especially if you know you are going to require donor eggs, donor sperm, a donor embryo or a surrogate, an infertility consultant may be worthwhile. It can be helpful to have someone with no financial bias offer advice.

How much of an investment? It depends. Fees range from $1,200 to $8,000, depending on what you need. Mindy Berkson, a Chicago-based infertility consultant, explains, "We establish a master plan to tackle the pathway to parenthood, taking into consideration emotional tolerances, the total financial budget, time frames and parameters for treatment opportunities. This plan also includes identified milestones for changing treatment and taking other courses of action." A consultant should help create a treatment plan, assist in insurance and financial planning, and some offer third-party reproductive services, such as gestational surrogate matching.

Consultants may not be able to save you their fee, but they can offer a calm voice, someone you can talk to, and they may know who the best physician is for you, where the support groups are, and other resources. "We can be a port in the storm," explains Toni Siragusa, a financial planner with Lotus Blossom Consulting. "You may not have other people in your life to talk to about your test results or communication problems with your physician's office, and we are a better person to ask or to bounce ideas off of than someone in a chat room or someone's cousin who went through IVF five years ago. We are an open mind and an advocate for you in the way a physician's office can't be. And if you're in a collaborative cycle with an egg donor or surrogate, we know which agencies keep the intended parent's needs and concerns at the forefront, and which ones are careless enough to let cocaine users through. There are crappy agencies out there. We won't name them, but we will steer a client away from them."

A fertility coach is another paid professional who can provide assistance to those going through infertility. Similar to a life coach, a fertility coach helps you look forward during your treatments and keep an optimistic attitude. Linda Tillman, PhD, explains, "I think of myself as the person behind my client when she hits emotional roadblocks. It's my job as the coach to address the roadblocks and keep the person moving down the road." This can include weighing complicated options such as deciding on different treatments, choosing to take a break, pursuing adoption, or resolving to be a child-free family.

If this interests you, do the research and contact at least two or three you may want to work with and see if what they offer is better than what you can do yourself. Thanks to modern technology, both infertility consultants and coaches can work entirely by telephone and internet. If you have the money necessary to take advantage of their services, you can utilize them no matter where you live.

A World of Information at Your Fingertips

*"I probably spent about $500 the first month I got my diagnosis.
I bought every book I could find that was even remotely related,
subscribed to a fertility magazine, and bought whatever vitamins
the eighteen-year-old salesclerk at the health food store suggested. In
hindsight, I may have gone a little overboard. That alone would
have paid for an IUI cycle."*

—CHRISTINA

When we experience something as all-consuming as infertility, it is easy to feel starved for information. We want to know everything—what we are dealing with, how to fix it, and where to start. We have lots and lots of questions and crave answers, more answers than our health care providers alone can offer. Also, we want to be able to address our concerns at any time, even if it is two o'clock in the morning. There is a wealth of information available to you, but how do you decide what is most beneficial?

INFERTILITY ORGANIZATIONS

Organizations focusing on infertility are popping up all the time. There are more than 165 organizations that claim to provide information and resources about infertility. These include more general infertility organizations as well as ones addressing certain infertility-related diseases, diagnoses, and treatments. They also include nonprofit organizations, government agencies, and even some for-profit businesses.

These organizations can provide you with some good resources. Although most offer information and assistance for free, some take advantage of the situation and require you to shell out money, whether it's for membership or information. Successful organizations receive the majority of their funding through grants and donations. If someone requests money from you in exchange for basic information, look elsewhere. We guarantee someone else has exactly what you need for free.

Also, organizations that rely on the infertility industry for financial support are unable to provide fair and balanced information to consumers. Look for biases and be aware of whose best interest is being served.

WEBSITES AND THE INTERNET

Typing the word *infertility* into Google yields more than 14 million websites. And this doesn't even count trying other related terms such as ART, IVF, donor sperm, donor eggs, donor embryos, surrogacy, gestational carriers, and the like. When you are dealing with infertility and making decisions about what to do, the internet is a great place to start. It is easily accessible and, most important, it's free. Even if you don't have internet access at home, you can go to the local library for free access.

You can usually get a lot accomplished in a relatively short period by surfing the net. Nearly everyone has a website overflowing with information. The internet is the infertility community's most important marketing

WANT TO KNOW IF A HEALTH WEBSITE IS RELIABLE?

Check to see if it has the HON logo. Health on the Net Foundation is the leading organization promoting and guiding the presentation of useful and reliable online medical and health information. HON is a nonprofit, nongovernmental organization, accredited by the United Nations. For more information, and a list of accredited sites, go to http://www.hon.ch/.

tool. You can find out more information about your symptoms, diagnosis, and proposed treatment plan, as well as learn to carefully craft questions for your fertility clinic. It is also a good way to check out your fertility clinic and any other professionals you are paying to help you bring home a baby.

Online blogs can be another useful free source for gathering information. A blog is a website that offers up-to-date commentary or news on a particular subject. Because infertility is often such an isolating experience, people turn to blogs in order to vent and share information. Infertility blogs are tremendously popular, with some reporting hundreds of thousands of hits a week. Blogs can help you stay connected with others like you. You can share in others' stories, as well as exchange ideas and experiences about your particular situation. For a list of the top infertility blogs go to http://blogs .botw.org/Health/Reproductive_Health/Infertility/.

Because anyone can post just about anything on the internet, be wary if you come across something that seems too good to be true. Some experts estimate that at least half of the information on the internet is either false or incomplete. Here are a few questions to ask to ascertain the quality of the information you glean from the internet.

- Who created the site (i.e., qualifications and contact information)?
- Is the information accurate (i.e., includes all references, sources, and citations)?
- Is the information current?
- Is the information balanced and objective?
- Is the information complete (i.e., provides appropriate links to other sources)?

Unique Situations

Although infertility itself is nondiscriminatory, access to infertility treatments is. The majority of infertility patients fit a single description—white, middle-class, and married. While it is not impossible for those who do not quite fit this profile to find good treatment, it will require additional resources, including time and money.

Single Women

Our society is changing, and more single women are opting to try for a baby without a male partner. Unfortunately, some clinics continue to refuse to treat single women. One recent study reported of the 383 fertility clinics surveyed, 16 percent refused to provide IVF and IUIs to single women. Often clinics chalk this up to having such a high demand for services they must limit their treatments to married couples.

"I've always loved children. And I kept waiting and waiting and waiting for my Prince Charming. But he never showed up. So a few years ago, I decided to do it myself and have an IUI. Much to my shock, the doctor at my local fertility clinic refused to inseminate me as soon as I told him I wasn't married. I later found out this

same clinic refuses to do any type of infertility treatment for single women. If I had just brought a man—any man—with me to the clinic, he wouldn't have asked about my marital status. I'm sure I would have received treatment then. Some of my friends thought I was stupid for not having done this, but I don't want to lie to get health care."

—LYNDA

QUICK TIP!
When you check CDC and SART statistics, the report summaries for each clinic will indicate whether or not they treat single women.

A few women have turned to the law to fight this. They cite discrimination on the basis of marital status as well as legal protections for the disabled (the Supreme Court has held that infertility is a disability). But so far, the courts have not been consistent in their stance regarding single women and infertility treatments. To date, litigation has proven to be not only expensive, but also largely unsuccessful.

Instead, search for clinics that are supportive of single women from the beginning. This has been a tough decision already, and you shouldn't start off with an uphill battle. Expect exceptional care, no matter what your situation is.

GAYS AND LESBIANS

"Creating a baby is much harder than we ever expected. We are a committed and loving couple who wants very much to add a child to our family. But for lesbian couples getting pregnant requires the help of many people. In order to bring a baby into our family, we are depending on doctors, nurses, ultrasound techs, donors, donor labs, thermometers, UPS, CVS, First Response, Bank of America, MasterCard, and lawyers, just to name a few."

—TAMMY AND MAGGIE

Gays and lesbians also have difficulty locating fertility care and family-building options. In the United States, physicians have the right to choose their own patients as long as the patient is not in a medical emergency. This also extends to others involved in family building, such as adoption agencies, third-party reproduction agencies, counselors, attorneys, and pharmacists.

The fertility rights of gays and lesbians came into focus when in 2008 the California Supreme Court agreed to hear a case involving a lesbian who was kept from having infertility treatment due to her doctor's religion. In 2006, the ASRM, the leading voice in reproductive medicine, concluded that clinics have an ethical obligation to treat all requests for assisted reproduction equally, without regard to marital status or sexual orientation. Since this is simply a recommendation, clinics can ultimately decide for themselves whom to treat.

As a result, gays and lesbians must search for friendlier locales. Don't assume larger, more metropolitan areas are more liberal. Only the District of Columbia and eight states—California, Connecticut, Illinois, Massachusetts, New Jersey, New York, Pennsylvania, and Vermont—allow same-sex couples to complete second-parent adoptions, providing more opportunities for family building. For more information about gay- and lesbian-friendly clinics and agencies, talk to other same-sex couples or contact your local gay and lesbian organizations and ask for information about family building.

FAMILIES OF COLOR

Infertility among people of color has rarely been seen as an issue of concern within our society. Limited access to information and treatment, as well as costs, has significantly impacted the way people of color view options related to infertility. Although 44 percent of women facing infertility will seek some type of infertility treatment, only 31 percent of women of color will do so.

How does this affect your finances? Because the majority of infertility patients are Caucasian, the infertility industry clearly caters to this demographic. For example, most research about infertility causes, diagnoses, and treatments has not included men and women of color. As a result, we are still unclear as to how success rates may differ according to race and ethnicity. You are going to have to look at statistics with an added layer of scrutiny.

Additionally, for third-party reproduction, there is less access to donors and gestational carriers of various racial and ethnic backgrounds. If you desire a donor or gestational carrier of a certain race or ethnicity, you will have to search harder, which costs more in time and in money. Contact several third-party reproduction agencies about the make-up of their donor and gestational carrier lists, locate agencies that focus on maintaining a more diverse pool of potential donors or gestational carriers, or take steps to locate a donor or gestational carrier yourself.

The Most Important Team Member: *You!*

Never underestimate your power. You are your own best advocate, and you can make things happen no matter where your infertility journey takes you. Most important, don't be bullied. Keep the lines of communication open—with your doctor, with your partner, and with yourself. We all have moments of anger and frustration, but stay in control and be vocal about what you want and need.

Want to Do Your Homework?
If you are interested in the latest research in infertility, check out MedlinePlus. It's technical, but you'll find medical journal articles, extensive information about drugs, an illustrated medical encyclopedia, and interactive patient tutorials: http://www.nlm.nih.gov/medlineplus/.

Consider infertility treatment as a part-time job with a delayed payoff. Making lifestyle changes, weighing financial decisions, and perusing research articles and online blogs take time and energy—and that's without going to the doctor! Taking care of yourself during this journey doesn't mean adding one more job to an already full plate. Instead, without apology, turn down any extra responsibilities and commitments to focus on your health and your relationships.

Being an active participant in your infertility treatment helps you best deal with the trials and tribulations of the infertility roller coaster. Also, all of these suggestions are free—an ideal price to pay for something that just might have an impact after all.

Five Things You Can Do Right Now

1. With your clinic short list in hand, research the fertility specialists' credentials.
2. Verify the labs' certifications and the embryologists' experience and training.
3. Ask if your potential clinics offer mental health resources.
4. Consider if any complementary therapy interests you and begin re-searching.
5. Find local and/or online support groups.

Chapter 5

So Many Choices:
Start a Treatment Plan

*"The Great Big Fertility Ride begins the day I am talking with
my family doctor about how my partner and I can't seem to get
pregnant. He seems casual about this, we haven't been trying
consistently, my partner goes away a fair bit, blah blah. But then I
mention that we have been together for ten years and that our chief
form of contraception in all that time has been the withdrawal
method. And that I'm thirty-five. His face clouds, he sucks in
oxygen, great big red lights start flashing around the room, an
alarm goes off, and a large neon clock descends from the ceiling and
begins to monster me with its incessant tick. 'Ah,' says the doctor, 'in
that case I think you better see someone and have some . . . tests.'"*
—Annie

Egg + Sperm = Baby, right? When this doesn't work, there is no quick
and easy route. Instead, we are faced with a long, convoluted journey with
choices at every turn. There are no simple answers here, because what works
for one person does not necessarily work for someone else. And you can't
predict with certainty what will work for you and when.

Fertility treatments seem to involve a lot of wait and see. With limited
resources, we can afford only so much experimentation and downtime.
Waiting to find out if something will work is frustrating when all you want
is a baby *now*.

We will provide you with information to help you make best choices
about your treatment options. There isn't a definitive right or wrong way of
doing things to get pregnant. Armed with a more thorough understanding
about your treatment options—what they involve, why they are recommended, and why they might work for you—you can start to regain some

control over your fertility. Ask the right questions and explore the most effective options, and protect your time and money.

Pretreatment Necessities

By the time you enter the door of the fertility clinic, your testing has already started. Ideally, your gynecologist or primary care physician has already covered the basics and checked the overall health of you and your partner for any underlying conditions that might be affecting your fertility (such as tumors, high blood pressure, diabetes, or an infection). Both partners will also have to be screened for sexually transmitted infections. In fact, sexually transmitted infections (even past infections), such as chlamydia, gonorrhea, syphilis, genital warts, and herpes, are a leading cause of infertility. For women, basic hormone levels need to be checked as well.

Possible Lab Tests for Both Women and Their Male Partners

TEST	AVERAGE COST PER TEST
Chlamydia and gonorrhea	$100
Hepatitis A	$50
Hepatitis B	$50
Hepatitis C	$100
HIV	$100–$200
Syphilis	$50
Human papilloma virus (HPV): women only	$100
Herpes	$140
Trichomoniasis	$5
Cholesterol	$50
Rubella	$50

Basic Hormone Labs for Women

	OPTIMAL TESTING TIME	WHAT IS IT TESTING?	AVERAGE COST PER TEST
Luteinizing Hormone (LH)	Cycle Day 3	Ovulation	$75
Follicle Stimulating Hormone (FSH)	Cycle Day 3 and Cycle Day 10	Ovarian function and onset of menopause	$75
Anti-Mullerian Hormone (AMH), Inhibin B, and FSH	Cycle Day 3	Ovarian reserve	$350
Estradiol (E2)	Cycle Day 3 and Cycle Day 10	Ability to maintain a healthy uterine lining	$75
Progesterone	7 Days Postovulation	Indicator of ovulation and necessary to support pregnancy	$75
Prolactin	Before a Breast Exam	A pituitary gland tumor that can prevent ovulation	$75
Thyroid Stimulating Hormone (TSH)	Anytime	A thyroid condition that can affect fertility	$50
Testosterone	Anytime	Presence of PCOS, which can affect fertility	$50–$200

If these tests have not been completed, see which ones can be done before you go to your fertility doctor. Often certain tests and diagnostics will be covered if ordered by a gynecologist or primary care physician, but not by a fertility specialist. This comes down to insurance coding (see chapter 7 for more details). Many of these test results are not limited to fertility. So if your gynecologist orders them and codes them under a "general" woman's health code, they are usually covered. If it appears they are being done solely for infertility-related reasons, then you might be out of luck. Just seeing a fertility specialist and having that doctor order the tests lets the cat out of the bag. Talk about this with your doctor and insurance company *before* any tests are ordered.

Your gynecologist or primary care physician may suggest waiting for the specialist, but most doctors are sympathetic to the limitations of insurance coverage and will accommodate you. In either case, before you move forward, call your local fertility clinic and ask which tests it recommends and what its fees for them are. Compare this with what your gynecologist or primary care physician can provide as well as what your insurance covers.

You can save money on these tests. Fees for lab work vary widely, so compare prices among different labs and clinics. Clinics like Planned Parenthood often offer tests for sexually transmitted infections for free or at a reduced cost. To accurately compare prices, get the Current Procedural Terminology (or CPT) code from the health care provider prescribing the test. The CPT code is a universally accepted number that corresponds to all billable tests and diagnostics, such as an MRI or lab test. Knowing these codes can help you obtain price quotes from several different providers in your area. To find out CPT codes, use the American Medical Association's free and easy-to-use CPT code search engine at www.ama-assn.org.

Some consumer-driven independent labs offer even deeper savings. Once you know which tests you need, you can go to one of their local collection sites to have your blood drawn. Some will even send a trained phlebotomist to your home or workplace to take the blood sample. The vials then get mailed to independent labs that can conduct more than fifteen hundred different tests. The lab will then mail the confidential results directly to both you and your doctor. While you should verify with your doctor about the reliability of using an outside lab, most of these independent labs state they use the same testing partners as physicians and hospitals.

Men, if you haven't already submitted to the oh-so-fun semen analysis, it's time. Fertility diagnoses need to start with the male partner, since over one-third of couples are diagnosed with male-factor problems. Luckily, this test is relatively quick and easy. Shop around, but semen analysis will set you back between $100 and $300. While some clinics and specialty labs offer more "assistance" in terms of comfortable rooms, magazines, and videos, your costs are going to be higher here. To save money, go to the cheapest lab's restroom and bring your own reading material or imagination.

Test results must be current. If it's been over a year, lab results won't count and will need to be repeated. Once you have done all you can do with your primary care provider or gynecologist, get copies of all your medical records to take with you to the fertility clinic. Review these records until you understand every test result and what it means. This is an important step in maintaining control over your course of treatment.

Your fertility specialist may request more tests at your first visit. Don't blindly say yes to everything he suggests. Bring all your lab results and medical records with you and review them carefully with your fertility specialist. Ask about the results of each test and how they will help in determining an effective treatment plan. Take notes to ensure the new tests being ordered are not duplications. If he insists these tests be done again, ask for an explanation.

LEGITIMATE REASONS FOR REPEATING LAB TESTS

- The test results are too old.

- The results are inconclusive.

- The particular lab may be known for certain errors.

- Tests could have been done at the wrong time in your cycle.

"We just like to do these tests ourselves to be sure" is not a valid response. If your insurance company covers these costs, then little harm is done, but you may still have to pay a percentage in terms of a deductible or copay. Regardless of who's footing the bill, it is completely reasonable to question the need for certain tests and negotiate a less expensive compromise.

Schedule your initial appointment with your fertility specialist during the first week of your cycle so baseline hormone levels can be checked. If this isn't done, you'll have to come back again, resulting in more costs. Bring in that BBT chart you've been keeping so your doctor can help you determine when and if you have been ovulating. Since 40 percent of infertility problems have to do with an ovulation disorder, BBT charts can be an important tool. If it appears you are ovulating regularly, you can move on to other tests more quickly.

Be honest with your fertility specialist. He is going to ask you personal questions, such as your cycle length, how regular your cycle is, if you have PMS, if you can tell when you are ovulating, and if you have painful periods. Even worse, your sex life is on display for all to hear. You get to talk about frequency, timing, use of lubricants, orgasms, and positions.

You and your partner will be asked if you have ever been pregnant or created a pregnancy, even ones aborted or miscarried. You will be asked about exposure to health hazards and lifestyle factors, including alcohol and drug use. All of these things could have a bearing on your fertility. As embarrassing as it may be, be completely honest. By providing as much information as possible, you can move forward without unnecessary testing and with a more appropriate and potentially more effective treatment plan.

Keep track of the tests you need and how they are covered under your insurance plan to maximize your benefits. By being an educated consumer early on, learning to question, and "shopping around" for these initial tests, you can start saving money now.

More Extensive Testing

Once these initial tests have been completed, it's time to move on to more specialized testing at your fertility clinic. You won't need every test offered. There is room to negotiate. Ask questions to understand exactly *why* you need these particular tests. You might be able to talk your health care provider into some lower-cost alternatives.

Some of the additional tests your fertility specialist might recommend include:

Clomid Challenge Test

A Clomid challenge test checks for ovarian reserve, or the amount of eggs you have. This information aids in determining your potential response to injectable fertility medications. In total, this test averages $500. If you might have low ovarian reserve or you might have difficulty responding to the fertility medications (i.e., you are older or have already experienced symptoms of early menopause), consider taking this test. In the end, $500 is cheaper than jumping right into a $15,000 IVF cycle that might not work.

Postcoital Test

A postcoital test really is the "immediately after you have had sex" test. After sex, you rush into the doctor's office so they can take a swab of the cervix (much like a Pap test) to see if the sperm can penetrate and survive in the cervical mucus. Due to frequent false or inconclusive results, research suggests this test does not provide much useful information, and you can decide not to have it done. At $125 per test, don't waste your money.

Ultrasound Exams

Your fertility specialist wants to look at your reproductive organs with the transvaginal ultrasound. There is no way around this one—it provides a wealth of information as to what's happening with your ovaries and uterus. You will definitely need ultrasounds with each new cycle. But at $200 to $300 each, how many of these do you need? Since they are quick and easy to do, doctors use them often. Remind your doctor how much you are paying for each one so they can be scheduled on the correct days of your cycle. Ask what he or she is looking for and why it must be done. Even one less ultrasound can save you a few hundred dollars.

Endometrial Biopsy

A small sample of the uterine lining is obtained and examined under a microscope for abnormalities, giving information about whether or not the uterus can support a pregnancy. This test typically costs around $300 and should be performed only if you have signs of a luteal phase defect (meaning the lining of your uterus isn't thick enough to support a pregnancy), such as a short cycle or low levels of progesterone.

Hysterosalpingogram (HSG)

Performed by a trained radiologist, a hysterosalpingogram is an x-ray procedure to examine your fallopian tubes for blockages. After all, that little egg needs to be able to make its way out of the ovary and down the fallopian tubes to get fertilized. About 30 percent of women undergoing ARTs have some type of tubal problem. At over $1,000 per HSG, you need this test only if you fall into this category, including those with endometriosis or previous pelvic surgery that could have resulted in scar tissue.

Sonohysterogram/Saline Ultrasound

A sonohysterogram (also called a saline ultrasound) is often better tolerated than a traditional HSG and can be performed in the doctor's office. With this procedure, saline is injected into the uterus while an ultrasound is being performed. At less than $1,000, this test is used to look for polyps, fibroids, and other uterine abnormalities getting in the way of fertility. However, this test is not as useful for checking to see if your tubes are open.

Hysteroscopy

A hysteroscopy provides a way for your physician to look inside your uterus. This tool helps a physician diagnose or treat a uterine problem. It can be especially useful for women who are at risk for polyps, scar tissue, or intrauterine fibroids that may be causes for their infertility. A hysteroscope is a thin, telescopelike instrument that is inserted into the uterus through the vagina and cervix. Hysteroscopy is a minor outpatient surgery. It can be performed with local, regional, or general anesthesia. It takes about thirty minutes, and can cost anywhere from $750 to $4,000, depending on the extent of the procedure, the surgical setting, and the anesthesia used. Because it is considered surgery, it should fall under your insurance coverage.

Laparoscopy

A laparoscopy can further explore or correct any defects with your uterus and fallopian tubes, including endometriosis, lesions, or scar tissue. Because of the cost and invasive nature, it should not be routine procedure. If you clearly have an ovulation problem or a severe sperm defect, then a laparoscopy isn't going to help you conceive.

Traditionally, laparoscopy has been performed in the hospital, but a few physicians perform it in their offices. The office is cheaper—it weighs in at about $1,500 compared to $2,000 to $10,000 in the hospital. The main advantage to performing laparoscopy in an office setting is reduced cost. If you go the hospital route, problems can generally be corrected while you are under general anesthesia, lessening the need for additional surgeries.

Because this is surgery, it will very likely be covered by insurance. Check your insurance carefully on this one. Some policies will cover it only if performed by a gynecologist and not by a fertility specialist.

Too Much Information

Is there such a thing as too much information? When it comes to infertility testing, sometimes the answer is yes. If you are paying for all your treatments yourself, the results of certain tests can help guide you toward the most effective treatments for your money. If you have some insurance coverage for treatment, infertility testing may be used to deny you coverage. For instance, some insurance plans do not pay for IVF for women who have high FSH levels or a failed Clomid challenge test. Since there is such a slim chance IVF will work, they don't want to foot the bill. Before you undergo any of these more extensive tests, ask your doctor about any implications of the results. There might be other ways to get the same information without jeopardizing your right to attempt certain treatments.

On Our Way: Initial Treatment Options

You should be closer to finding out what the problem is now. If not, you're in good company, since at least 10 percent of patients fall into the category of "unexplained infertility." Regardless, now it's time to move on to some more active treatment options. Next in line is usually some variation of intrauterine insemination (IUI), formerly known as "artificial insemination." Success rates for bringing home a baby vary, ranging from 6 percent to 26 percent depending on how many follicles (or eggs) are produced. While it is relatively low-tech, an IUI works better than just having intercourse on your own. For women over forty, women with elevated FSH levels, or when sperm are compromised in number or function, success rates with IUIs are lower and may not be worth your time and money. You might be better off moving quickly to IVF. How do you know what to do and when? Let's look at some of the specifics related to IUIs.

Intrauterine Insemination (IUI)

An IUI involves placing washed sperm (a $100 procedure that separates the sperm from the rest of the seminal fluid and increases the chance for success) directly into the uterus through a small catheter at ovulation. By bypassing the cervix, more sperm are placed in the uterus than would naturally get there. Typical costs for a "natural" cycle IUI (without the use of any fertility meds) range from $300 to $700. Monitoring ovulation through blood tests (about $85-$100 per test) and transvaginal ultrasounds (about $300 per test) add to your fees. Overall, you are looking at about $1,000 to $2,000 per basic IUI attempt.

What if your partner's sperm is not up to par? Some specialists say you need only about 1 million washed sperm to try IUI. Higher success rates are associated with washed counts over 20 million to 30 million. Counts of at least 10 million offer the most cost-effectiveness for IUI, since there is a good overall chance for success. There is a significant reduction in pregnancy rates when the count is lower than 10 million. For counts lower than 5 million, look at other options with better odds.

MEDICATED IUI CYCLES

Ovulation is the key to the success of IUI. To produce more good-quality follicles and eventually eggs to mix with that sperm, IUI can be combined with ovulation-induction medications. Often clomiphene citrate is used with IUI and adds another $60 to $150 to the cost per attempt, depending on the dosage prescribed.

If clomiphene citrate fails, you may move on to the higher priced injectable medications (also called gonadotropins). Women over thirty-five years of age with no known ovulation problems are sometimes encouraged to skip the clomiphene citrate and proceed more aggressively to gonadotropin treatment. These gonadotropins cost about $100 per ampule and you will need 10 to 40 ampules per cycle plus about $60 for a shot of hCG to trigger ovulation. The grand total for the injectable medications can vary from $400 to $3,000 per attempt, on top of the $1,000 to $2,000 IUI procedure costs.

A major downside of medicated IUIs is the risk of multiple births. Women who get pregnant using injectables and IUI have a 10 percent to 15 percent chance of carrying multiples (many of which are triplets or higher). With these types of potent medications, it is likely you will release more eggs, and there is no way to predict or control how many will get fertilized. From a financial standpoint, this can be a big gamble if you are already struggling with money. Understand the risks and have a well-thought-out plan to deal with this situation if it arises.

How many times do you try IUI? It depends on what you can afford and what medications you are using. Research suggests trying three to four IUIs on clomiphene citrate before moving on to injectables, then attempt three to four cycles on injectables. If you don't have success after four good ovulatory cycles on injectables with well-timed IUI, it's time to start considering other alternatives such as IVF or egg donation.

Some clinics opt to do an IUI, wait a day, then do a second IUI. Research doesn't prove it's an effective use of money. If you've got good follicles, a trigger shot, and a well-timed insemination, then you're set. A second IUI in the same cycle does not increase your odds enough to justify the added cost.

DONOR SPERM

What if you don't have a willing male partner with good quality sperm? Investigate some independent sperm banks, since most fertility clinics do not work directly with sperm donors.

Donor sperm available in the United States is collected and processed by a relatively small number of sperm banks. You can also purchase sperm from banks located overseas as well and have it shipped here. As you can imagine, sperm fees vary among sperm banks, so be a smart shopper. In general, fees average $200 to $600 per vial of sperm.

Some sperm banks, particularly larger ones, have very complicated fee structures. Some sperm banks nickel and dime you, charging you at every turn—whether it's for a donor consultation (to help you pick a donor), photo matching (where you provide a photo of your partner, and they find a donor with similar appearance), and genetic consultations. Choosing an open donor (or one willing to have his identity revealed) can be an additional cost. You can also pay extra for detailed profiles, genetic and health information, baby photos, video- or audiotaped interviews, psychological profiles, and handwritten essays. It adds up and can easily exceed the original $200 to $600 estimate, depending on how many extras you buy. Some banks require a membership fee to their bank before they will even let you start the process.

> *"We used every available penny to order three vials of donor sperm . . . a whopping $1,095. We knew our clinic would charge a storage fee, but we assumed it would be like our other clinic, which billed for the storage. I received a call a few hours ago that they need*

the payment before the little swimmers arrive! Yikes! I started
calling to get balance information on our credit cards—not enough
available credit—rechecked our checking account—damn near
zero—and for a moment considered selling one of my kidneys on
the black market. How much can you get for a kidney nowadays?"
—Dana

If you want a more desirable donor, such as one with an advanced degree or certain characteristics, you will most certainly pay more. Some sperm banks advertise a special section of doctorate or professional donors (such as physicians, lawyers, and PhDs). There is no research to suggest choosing one of these types of donors will improve your child's health, intellect, or emotional intelligence, so save your money.

In general, semen specimens are usually sold in 1.2 cc vials or units. You need at least one unit for a single insemination. While it usually costs a few hundred dollars, the fees vary depending on how you are going to use it: for intracervical insemination (ICI), intrauterine insemination (IUI), or in vitro fertilization (IVF). IUI is usually the most expensive, and IVF is the cheapest. You can also order the sperm prewashed, which typically costs about $50 to $150 more, or you can wait to have it washed at your fertility clinic before the IUI or IVF. Check with your fertility clinic so you don't pay to have it double-washed.

Shipping fees vary and depend on where you want it shipped. The costs of shipping range from free to more than $200, depending on where it must be shipped, how soon you want it, whether you need Saturday delivery, and so on. It must be carefully packed in dry ice or liquid nitrogen. Semen remains viable for up to a week shipped in liquid nitrogen, but only a few days with dry ice. Sperm banks require a refundable tank deposit in case you lose or damage the storage/shipping tank. Some even charge a daily rental fee if you are late returning the tank. If the sperm bank is local, you can avoid shipping charges by picking up the vials yourself.

You might consider purchasing more sperm than you need for a single IUI. This is especially important if you have your sights set on a specific donor and don't want to go through the selection process again if the first IUI doesn't work. Likewise, if you would like to have the option of creating full genetic siblings, you will need additional sperm from that donor as well.

Because donors can stop donating at any time, you may choose to buy out your donor's current sperm supply. Remember, you'll have to buy the sperm and pay to have it stored. No, your freezer is not an option. What if you end up not using all your vials? Ask about their return policy or if you can donate them to another family.

Sample Sperm Bank Charges

ANONYMOUS DONORS

Premium ICI (Intracervical Insemination)	$350
Premium IUI (Intrauterine Insemination)	$420
ART (IVF)	$300

OPEN DONORS

Premium ICI (Intracervical Insemination)	$440
Premium IUI (Intrauterine Insemination)	$520
ART (IVF)	$400

DONOR INFORMATION

Short Donor Profile	Free
Staff Impressions Report	Free
Donor Essay	Free
Short Donor Profile (via fax)	$5
Long Donor Profile	$16
Donor Audio Interview	$26
Donor Baby Photo	$21
Facial Features Report	$13

DELIVERY AND SHIPPING FEES

Mail: Up to 3 items	$5
Mail: 4 or more items	$10
FedEx: Letter	$25
FedEx: Package	$30
FedEx: Saturday Delivery	Add $10

CONSULTATION SERVICES

Donor Photo Matching	
1 to 6 Donors	$60
7 to 12 Donors	$120
Phone Donor Selection Consultation (Includes: Initial phone interview, photo matching, half hour with a genetic counselor, call back with selection results, and detailed information for up to two donors)	$300
In-house Donor Selection Consultation (Includes: Initial phone interview, photo matching, half hour with a genetic counselor, call back with selection results, and detailed information for up to two donors)	$500
Genetic Counselor Consultation	$90 per hour

A few fertility clinics have developed strong relationships or partnerships with certain sperm donor agencies. These clinics may require you to go through these donor programs, maximizing profits for both them and the donor agency. Because you are a captive audience here, your choices will be limited and you will have fewer opportunities for negotiation or cost savings. In any case, clarify the protocols for both the sperm bank and your clinic in terms of handling, delivering, storing, and using the donated sperm. Since there are several entities involved, everyone needs to be on the same page.

Some women opt for finding their own donors, such as a close friend or family member. This isn't free, either. No matter how well you know this person, he still needs to be tested so you have general medical information and screening for infectious diseases, including sexually transmitted infections and HIV, not to mention counseling to ensure he understands the ramifications of donating sperm. Before you begin, get approval from your clinic about using a known sperm donor, because many clinics will refuse to work with known sperm donors.

If you are using donor sperm and have no indications of any infertility issues, then you might be privy to some very cost-effective shortcuts. For instance, you don't need to visit an official fertility clinic to be inseminated with donor sperm. Some gynecologists will perform an IUI in their office, and some independent clinics specialize in inseminating otherwise fertile women with donor sperm.

Then there is the proverbial "turkey baster" method, or more technically called intracervical insemination (ICI). With ICI, sperm is deposited directly into your cervix and is far less expensive then IUI, which places the sperm into the uterus. Women who are typically fertile, have no underlying problems with their reproductive organs, and are ovulating regularly might want to consider ICI as a less expensive alternative. As with IUI, ICI must be timed perfectly to correspond with ovulation to be successful. You must know your body well enough to anticipate ovulation or be willing to pay for ovulation monitoring.

ICI is usually performed in a clinic, although some women opt to do this in the privacy of their own homes (which of course lessens expenses even more). If your state and sperm bank allow, frozen sperm can be shipped directly to you. You then insert the sperm into the vagina similar to what would occur during intercourse. Talk to a trained health care provider first about the proper techniques because it can be dangerous if not done properly. And talk to the sperm bank or a reproductive attorney to find out if you live in a state governed by strict laws forbidding anyone other than a physician from doing inseminations.

Five Things You Can Do Right Now

1. Create a menstrual cycle diary. Start charting when your periods start and end, what your symptoms were, and if your flow was unusually light or heavy.
2. Bring your BBT chart, medical history, and any past records from your gynecologist.
3. Arrive early to fill out paperwork completely and accurately. If you can, have it mailed, so you can fill it out when you have more time.
4. Communicate with your insurance company *before* your visit about what will be covered during the visit.
5. Be prepared and focused. What do you want to happen during the appointment?

Chapter 6

Expecting the Unexpected:
The Move to Assisted Reproductive Technology (ART)

Assisted Reproductive Technologies (ARTs) include all fertility treatments in which both eggs and sperm are handled in a lab setting. ARTs involve surgically removing eggs from a woman's body, combining them with sperm in a petri dish for fertilization, and transferring them to a woman's body or freezing them for transfer at a later date. It is far from an exact science, with variations tailored to each woman's unique conditions. Although almost one in every three ARTs results in the birth of a baby, ART is invasive and expensive. When lower-tech treatments don't work, fertility specialists recommend moving on to some form of assisted reproductive technology. Reasons specialists may recommend ARTs include:

- Blocked fallopian tubes
- Male-factor issues
- Endometriosis
- Diminished ovarian reserve
- Advanced maternal age
- Loss of ovarian function
- Unexplained infertility

We'll look at each of the different forms of ART in turn.

In Vitro Fertilization (IVF)

IVF is by far the most common ART performed and has been available since the mid-1970s. With IVF, your eggs are combined with your partner's (or donor's) sperm in a lab. Once fertilization occurs, the resulting embryos develop for 3 to 5 days before being placed in your uterus. Some estimate that 1 percent to 3 percent of all babies born are the result of IVF. Success rates average around 40 percent, but can range from 16 percent to over 66 percent, depending on clinic quality, age of patient, and fertility history.

Not every cycle of IVF is the same, and there are a few variations of IVF, each of which comes with a different price tag. As a result, there may be a few opportunities to negotiate cost savings without sacrificing quality of care.

Costs for a basic IVF cycle vary greatly, from about $6,000 to over $25,000, not including medications. The vast majority of clinics fall somewhere in the $10,000-to-$15,000 range, plus medications, for a single attempt. All clinics will defend their price list, but with such a wide variation, there is wiggle room at most of these clinics.

There is no overall standard for exact procedures and costs for IVF. Every fertility specialist has a slightly different approach, although there are two basic protocols for conventional IVF—the long and the short.

In the long protocol, which is the most popular, drugs are given in a nasal spray or injections to stop the ovaries and throw the woman into a temporary menopause, otherwise known as *down regulation*. Then injections of another drug are given every day for a week and a half to stimulate the ovaries to produce many eggs. Finally, a third drug is injected to make the eggs ripen, getting them ready for egg collection. The eggs are then retrieved, fertilized in the lab, and transferred back into the uterus.

AVERAGE IVF COSTS

- Clinic fees, including office visits, exams, and monitoring: $2,000 to $3,000

- Egg retrieval: $2,000 to $4,000

- Embryo lab charges: $2,000 to $5,000

- Embryo transfer: $1,000

- Medication costs: $2,000 to $6,000

The short protocol (also known as low-stim, minimal stimulation intermediate protocol, the mild approach, or a mini-IVF) keeps your body as close to the natural state as possible by using less medication. A completely natural, or unmedicated, cycle avoids the use of ovarian stimulation drugs altogether. Short protocols are matched to the woman's natural cycle, allowing for significantly lower medication costs and making this option about 20 percent to 25 percent less expensive than the more aggressive regular IVF. It also takes less time—four weeks compared to six for conventional IVF.

Because this approach is much cheaper, more cycles can be done for the same money. For women under thirty-six, the success rates of the short protocol are good. And for older women and those who respond poorly to drug stimulation, they can sometimes be better. Those with just tubal problems or male-factor infertility are usually good candidates for the short protocol as well.

A disadvantage of the minimal stimulation protocol is that often (some suggest at least 20 percent to 30 percent of the time) cycles are canceled because ovulation occurs too early and the window for egg retrieval is missed. Also, fewer eggs (3 to 4 eggs if you are lucky) are produced than in standard IVF (10 to 20 eggs). This creates a reduced chance of producing extra embryos for freezing and use in a future cycle. This type of protocol is not routinely recommended, but for those who cannot afford standard IVF, minimal stimulation IVF may be worth considering.

Other Ways to Lower Costs

Ask about options for anesthesia during egg retrieval. There is a big cost difference between using general anesthesia versus twilight sleep or a simple sedative. Very few physicians are willing to do this, but some are open to forgoing general anesthesia and give a local so you can save more than $500. Ask about cycle monitoring and office visits. With each ultrasound costing about $300 and multiple office visit fees, speak up and ensure you are receiving the best medical care in the most efficient manner. Since most have to pay for this completely out of pocket, fertility clinics cannot assume we have no financial limits when scheduling exams and testing.

There are also hidden costs associated with IVF. For instance, IVF cycles can be canceled due to low response to the medications. You are still responsible for the costs incurred, so know what you are responsible for before you start down the path of IVF. Costs can also vary depending on age or fertility history. Women who are over thirty-five or who have had several failed IVF attempts in the past might be subjected to higher prices for similar services. Don't forget all those missed days of work and travel costs to and from the clinic nearly every day; they add up and leave you less money to try again.

Should You Fast-Track IVF?

For many women, an intrauterine insemination, or IUI (which we discussed in chapter 5), is a logical first step before trying a more rigorous (and more expensive) cycle of IVF treatment. At $1,000 to $2,000 per attempt, IUI is one of the cheapest infertility treatments available. To maximize the cost effectiveness, you must be a good candidate for IUI. You need to know you are ovulating, you do not have a serious male-factor problem, and everything seems to be in good working order otherwise. If not, you might want to consider other options earlier in the game.

However, researchers have recently begun to encourage certain women to skip multiple rounds of IUI and go straight to IVF, saving them both time and money. Also, because of the unpredictable risk of dangerous multiple births associated with medicated IUIs, some fertility clinics have started skipping IUIs and going straight to IVF more often as well. Since with an IVF, doctors are able to control how many embryos are transferred back, it brings the risk of higher-order multiples down to a somewhat more manageable 2 percent to 4 percent (but still way up from about 1 in 7,000 for the general population).

A 2007 study conducted by Dr. Richard Reindollar and colleagues concluded that while ultimate success rates were similar between women who used the conventional treatment method and those opting for the "fast-track" IVF protocol, the fast-track women had a 40 percent better chance of achieving pregnancy in the first year. Translated into dollars, women who were fast tracked into IVF got pregnant about three months faster and spent about $10,000 less than their counterparts following the conventional protocol. If you think you might be an appropriate candidate, you might want to inquire about skipping the multiple IUIs. However, experts are still unsure whether or not this fast-track option is a wise decision for all. And some insurance companies require you to attempt a certain number of IUIs first before moving on to IVF.

Third-Party or Collaborative Reproduction

"It takes a village . . ." takes on a new meaning when it comes to ARTs. For some women and couples, a little more help is needed in creating a new life. With this help comes an additional cost. It is difficult to ascertain the cost-effectiveness of third-party reproduction. Although third-party reproduction includes some of the most expensive infertility treatments, it also provides the opportunity to have a child a couple would never have had otherwise. It's hard to place a price tag on this.

Third-party, or "collaborative," reproduction typically consists of donor eggs, donor embryos, and/or surrogacy. These technologies include the different aspects of IVF (ovarian stimulation, egg retrieval, fertilization, and embryo transfer) plus the costs associated with the donor and/or surrogate. No matter how you slice it, these are expensive options. Costs are expected to continue to rise because of new FDA regulations governing the handling, storage, and use of human reproductive tissue, including sperm, eggs, and embryos. But if you have the money, third-party reproduction can offer you a chance to have a baby that might not have been possible otherwise.

Egg Donation

Egg donation creates an opportunity for at least 15,000 women a year to build their families. If your goal is simply to have a baby, and you have limited money, do not go through ten IVFs with your own eggs. It is more cost-effective to move on to donor eggs sooner than later. Egg donation involves the use of a donated egg (from a young and presumably very fertile woman) in an IVF cycle. For older women and those with high FSH levels, egg donation offers a much greater chance of success of having a live birth than IVF alone, in some cases greater than 50 percent. Sometimes women need to go through a few IVF cycles with their own eggs to gain a sense of closure. Ultimately, you will need to decide whether the desire to have a genetically related child is overshadowing your ability to bring home a baby as soon as possible.

Egg donation is more expensive than using your own eggs, but eggs from someone younger and not fertility-impaired will typically work better. Costs associated with egg donation range anywhere from $20,000 to $40,000. Many women exhaust a lot of time and money attempting IVF

AVERAGE EGG DONATION COSTS

- Clinic fees, including office visits, exams, testing, and monitoring for both the recipient and the donor: $2,000 to $6,000

- Psychological and medical screening for the donor: $1,000 to $2,000

- Egg retrieval from donor: $2,000 to $4,000

- Embryo lab charges: $2,000 to $5,000

- Embryo transfer to recipient: $500 to $750

- Egg administrative fees for clinic for the coordination of the donor match: $2,000 to $3,000

- Donor medications: $2,000 to $5,000

- Medications for the recipient: $500 to $1,000

- Fee to donor $5,000 to $10,000

- Additional costs for donor, including insurance, transportation, child care, et cetera: $1,000

when their chances with egg donation are significantly higher. This is an important consideration when designing your overall financial plan of action.

How can you save money here? Egg donation is incredibly expensive—there is no getting around this. Because these costs vary greatly among clinics, understand all of these costs before you start any egg donor cycle. The same questions pertaining to cost savings for IVF still apply here as well—ask about medication costs, maximizing the efficiency of office visits and testing, the use of anesthesia, and the possibility of canceled cycles.

Much of the high costs for donor egg cycles are related to the donor, so you have some options here. You can find a donor through your fertility clinics, or an independent egg donor agency, or you can find the donor yourself. From a strictly financial perspective, your fertility clinic offers the most continuity of care. Your clinic can coordinate your and your donor's needs in a more cost-effective manner. Since you are working with only one entity, you might have more opportunities to ask questions, negotiate costs, and even complain. The major drawback is that the egg donor coordinator makes the matching decisions and you have a handful of options—and maybe only one or two donors from which to choose.

Working with an independent party egg donor agency (also called an "egg broker") allows you more choices of egg donors and a quicker match. Agencies range from online catalogs to brick-and-mortar offices that work in conjunction with fertility clinics. Do your homework about these agencies to find one that is affordable as well as trustworthy and ethical. The ASRM publishes a list of egg donor agencies that agree to abide by strict ethical guidelines. You can find their list online at www.asrm.org.

Ask the agency about all the medical, legal, and financial arrangements regarding your egg donor. Most important, you need the agency to work well with your fertility clinic. This may include paying for additional travel costs for evaluations, exams, and treatments for you and your doctor, especially if you and your donor are located in different geographic areas. You will need to coordinate the eggs being retrieved from the donor, her eggs being fertilized with your partner's (or donor's) sperm, and the ultimate transfer of the embryos to your uterus. This type of coordination costs money.

All donor programs, whether clinic based or independent, must recruit donors. As a result, overhead costs are eventually transferred to you for the recruitment, evaluation, and care and keeping of these donors. If you wish to circumvent some of these costs and try to find the perfect donor on your own, these costs are replaced by other costs. For instance, you will need to pay for the advertisements to find the donor, provide access for the donor to contact you, set up the appropriate screenings and evaluations, hire an attorney to draw up contracts, and coordinate the treatment schedules between you and your donor. Consider finding your own donor if you are looking for a particular ethnic background, but know that it's tough to save money here.

Donor payment is another important financial consideration. Most clinics and agencies have a set donor payment price that ranges from $2,000 to $10,000, depending on clinic guidelines. If you select the donor on your own, you are able to negotiate your price a bit more. Typically somewhere between $5,000 and $10,000 is considered appropriate compensation for the approximately sixty hours over five to seven weeks the donor needs to complete the egg donation process.

Matching with a donor takes time, sometimes up to several months. To show you are serious, be prepared to fork over at least $1,000 just to be added to the wait list. If you are successful in finding a donor through this particular clinic or agency, the $1,000 will be applied to your treatment. If you change your mind or decide to go with another clinic or donor agency, you will forfeit this money. This minimizes the chance you will sign up with several donor programs just to see who gets to you the quickest.

You may be fortunate enough to have a family or friend who has offered to be an egg donor. This is not without its own complications. With a known donor, you might save on the donor payment, but you must still set aside some funds for extensive professional counseling on how to best adapt to this new relationship. As with any other donor, you will still be responsible for medical costs, screening expenses, and legal costs.

Embryo Donation

This is a long shot, but you may be able to receive someone else's donated embryos. After IVF, extra embryos are cryopreserved—frozen—for later use. If families decide against using these embryos themselves, destroying them, or donating them to research, they can donate them to another family. Only a few hundred babies have been born via donated embryos, largely because many families feel uncomfortable allowing another family to raise children they have created.

If you've exhausted all other options to have a genetic child, but still want to carry and give birth to a baby, talk to your clinic about the possibility of embryo donation. Your clinic will have information about any former patients who have decided to donate their embryos and make them available to other families. As with all forms of third-party reproduction, both the donor and recipient families should be screened and made aware of the psychological, moral, and legal implications of embryo donation.

The cost of embryo donation varies, but the total expenses average about one-third of the cost of a standard IVF cycle. The most expensive parts of an IVF cycle—fertility medications, egg retrieval, and fertilization and culture of the embryos—are already done.

In the embryo donation process, embryos are simply donated to another couple. Legally, only children who have been born can be adopted. But there are a number of independent embryo donation agencies that treat the donation of a frozen embryo as an actual adoption. This adds administrative costs and makes it less cost effective. If you use this type of agency, be prepared to pay an additional 25 percent to 50 percent for the application, administrative, assessment, and home study fees, often raising the price tag to a cost-prohibitive $20,000. Due to the controversy surrounding embryo adoption, it also may be hard to locate a fertility clinic that works with independent embryo adoption agencies. This means you will incur more travel costs.

AVERAGE EMBRYO "ADOPTION" COSTS

- Application fee: $200 to $300

- Home study and further assessments: $2,000 to $3,000

- Clinic facility fee: $1,000 to $2,000

- Additional administrative costs: $300 to $500

- Frozen embryo transfer: $750 to $1,000

- Embryology lab fees: $500 to $600

- Monitoring fee: $250

- Embryo shipping fee: $200

- Reimbursing the donor family for past storage fees for the embryos: $500

- Medical testing such as an STD rescreening: $500 to $1,000

The success rates of embryo donation are difficult to determine because much of the success depends on the lab conducting the original cryopreservation. Ask about the center and its experience with freezing embryos, the age of the woman who provided the eggs, the cause of the donating couple's infertility, quality of the embryos before they were frozen, developmental stage at which the embryos were frozen, and the number of frozen embryos available for donation. In general, success rates for this option will be lower if the woman who provided the eggs is older or if there were egg issues that contributed to her infertility. Obviously, if all your embryos do not survive the thaw, you will have fewer chances to make a baby.

SURROGATES AND GESTATIONAL CARRIERS

A traditional surrogate, or TS, donates her egg and loans her uterus to create a child. A gestational carrier, or GC, only loans her uterus. The egg can come from another donor or the intended mother. Couples can chose either based on their underlying problems and specific needs. While it's a more complicated, involved, and expensive procedure, most families opt to use a GC over a TS surrogate, so the surrogate has no genetic claim to the child.

Surrogacy costs are enormous. Because there are so many factors—eggs, uterus, and sperm—all coming from different sources, using a gestational carrier is often considered the most expensive of the ARTs and easily can top over $60,000. Some agencies warn you should anticipate over $100,000 in surrogacy-related expenses.

First, you must find a surrogate yourself, though your fertility clinic or through an independent surrogate agency. Most families choose to go through an independent surrogate program that specializes in helping families through the surrogacy experience medically, emotionally, and legally.

The reimbursement to the surrogate for her services is typically in the $13,000-to-$25,000 range. Additional payments are made in the cases of multiple births and/or a cesarean section. If you are working with a surrogacy agency, expect to pay about 50 percent to sign up with the agency, 25 percent of the fee when matched with the surrogate, and 25 percent after the first successful trimester of pregnancy. Since you will still need an egg donor, this will set you back another $20,000 to $40,000 for the entire egg donor procedure (unless you are using your own eggs, which would then make this part cost about the same as a traditional IVF).

Legal expenses are also critical to protect your interests. These typically include attorney fees for preparing documents for both before and after birth ($1,000 to $8,000), as well as court fees and costs ($500 to $800). Work with an experienced lawyer so you are well-protected; this is one place not to skimp. Experienced attorneys may also be able to help you locate a surrogate through his or her own network within the field. Since you have already chosen a professional you trust, if they know of an appropriate surrogate, this can save you a lot of time and money.

Using a surrogate is one of the most expensive family-building options. Little can be done to significantly reduce costs. You can utilize some of the

AVERAGE COSTS FOR FINDING
A GESTATIONAL CARRIER

- Advertising: at least $500

- GC's initial psychological evaluation: at least $500

- Medical insurance for the gestational carrier: $100 to $600 per month

- Life insurance policy for gestational carrier: $300

- Maternity clothing allowance: $500

- Costs associated with regular communication and contact: at least $200

- Payment to GC for lost wages: negotiated depending on job

- Gestational carrier's ongoing psychological counseling: varies

- Gestational carrier's independent lawyer's review of contracts and drafting of documents: $500 to $1,000

- Gestational carrier's medical testing: $500 to $1,000

- Maternity costs for doctor, delivery, prenatal care, and postnatal care: $10,000 to $20,000

cost-saving suggestions for both IVF and egg donation. Use a reputable surrogacy program with a good track record in terms of successful pregnancies and satisfied families and surrogates. Dig deep on internet bulletin boards and seek out as many people as you can who have experience with the agency. Ask for references and talk to them at length about their experiences.

Newer Developments

While we have covered the basics of infertility treatments, new techniques are becoming available that may increase your chances of bringing home a baby. They're not cheap either, so how do you know which ones are worth the added investment?

Micromanipulation

Intracytoplasmic sperm injection, more commonly known as ICSI (pronounced ick-see), is just a fancy way of saying "injecting a single sperm directly into an egg." Since technically you need only one sperm to fertilize an egg, men with male-factor infertility can now conceive a child. ICSI is done through the micromanipulation of the sperm and egg by a well-trained embryologist using special microscopes and tiny, specially designed needles. What began as treatment for male-factor infertility has become the fastest-growing infertility treatment. Today, clinics routinely use ICSI as part of all IVF cycles, and fertilization rates are high—about 60 percent to 85 percent of eggs are successfully fertilized with ICSI.

Is it worth the extra $1,000 to $1,500? For those with male-factor infertility, with unexplained infertility, or who are low responders who produce few eggs or eggs difficult to fertilize, absolutely. It's still too early to tell if it should be used in all cases of IVF. Despite popular beliefs, ICSI does not guarantee fertilization. Some research indicates that bypassing the simple biological tenet of "let the best sperm win," subpar sperm are being used to fertilize eggs, perhaps increasing the chances of passing along genetic abnormalities to the resulting children. And for right now, the overall baby take-home rates seem to be about the same for both ICSI and non-ICSI IVF cycles.

If you can't afford it or it's your first IVF, you don't have to do ICSI. If you are unsure, there are some cost-saving options. Some clinics that use ICSI frequently may be willing to provide some discounts in costs. A split ICSI-IVF cycle where only some of the eggs are fertilized with ICSI can also save a few hundred dollars.

Assisted hatching is another form of micromanipulation in which a small hole is made in the outer coating (or *zona*) that surrounds the egg. While success rates vary from clinic to clinic, this procedure may increase the chances of fertilization. Increased success is seen more often in women over the age of thirty-nine, with elevated FSH levels, several failed IVF cycles, and eggs with a thick outer coating. Assisted hatching adds about $500 to the cost of an IVF and the jury is still out on its cost-effectiveness.

The key to these types of micromanipulation procedures is the skill of your clinic's embryologist. Ask about the qualifications of the embryologist, his or her experience with these types of procedures, how often they are performed, and what the outcomes were. Ensure you are getting the most for your additional money.

GENETIC TESTING AND GENDER SELECTION

Preimplantation genetic diagnosis (PGD) allows the embryo to be tested for gender and certain genetic disorders a few days after fertilization, before it is transferred to the uterus. PGD does not help with either fertilization or implantation, and pregnancy rates are similar for embryos that underwent PGD as for those that did not. At $5,000, PGD is recommended only for families at risk for passing along genetic abnormalities to their offspring. It is still not widely used and is currently performed in only 4 percent of all IVF cycles. While some families with a history of genetic problems have tried getting insurance to cover it, we haven't heard of one yet that would. PGD can test for sixty diseases, including: cystic fibrosis, Down syndrome, Trisomy 21, Tay Sachs, Turner's syndrome, hemophilia A and B, Gaucher's disease, and sickle cell anemia. Some genetic diseases can occur in a child of a specific gender—PGD allows the identification of the embryo's sex so only unaffected ones will be transferred back.

PATIENTS WHO MIGHT BENEFIT FROM PGD

- Carriers of known genetic diseases

- Women over the age of thirty-eight

- Women who have had recurrent miscarriages

- Couples who have had previous aneuploid conceptions

- Women with three or more failed IVFs

For families interested in gender selection or family balancing, some fertility centers offer *sperm sorting*, a technique designed to increase the likelihood of conceiving a child of a particular gender. This is available at only a couple of select clinics; there's a $300 nonrefundable consultation fee just to discuss this option. The actual procedure costs $3,500 for one vial of semen, not including freezing, storage, or shipping fees. Frankly, if you can afford to pay $4,000 just to gender select, then put down this book before the rest of us get annoyed at you. Many clinics refuse to participate in any type of sex selection except for genetic issues.

Embryo Grading

There is no doubt that the ability to identify "good quality" embryos is increasing as our technology and understanding of embryo growth are improving. In general, embryos are assessed primarily by looking at cell number, cell regularity, and degree of fragmentation starting at day two of development. Embryos with higher cell numbers, more regular-appearing cells, and little or no fragmentation have a higher overall chance of implanting.

However, there are many other contributing factors regarding whether or not an embryo will be successful. There are many beautiful and healthy babies born by transferring low-grade embryos. Likewise, many cycles also fail after transferring perfect looking embryos.

In terms of making the most of your money, if you have made it this far in your fertility treatments, you might as well try to transfer the best looking embryos you have. After all, you aren't going to get any money back by canceling the cycle at this point. Grading embryos is not an exact science, and there are no universal guidelines to determine how good an embryo is. What looks poor to one embryologist might look fine to another. We say take the best embryos you have and go for it. You just never know which one is going to stick.

Timing of Transfer

Once the egg is fertilized and allowed to grow for a few days, you have a few choices in terms of the actual embryo transfer. First, the best quality embryos are selected by the lab for transfer. In the past, embryos have been transferred to the uterus at about 2 to 3 days. Today, embryos are able to grow in the lab until 5 days, when they become blastocysts. By this time, survival of the fittest comes into play; embryos that make it to the blastocyst stage have a greater likelihood of achieving a pregnancy. It's a catch-22 situation, though. By waiting until the fifth day, many embryos do not survive. Extra days sitting in the lab might not cost much more, but you could lose all your embryos, so talk with your fertility specialist to help you make the best decision.

"This was my fourth IVF. I always responded well to the meds, but the fertilized eggs never implanted. This cycle we decided to wait longer to transfer. On retrieval day they retrieved twenty-two mature eggs. Three days later they called and said nineteen had fertilized. At blastocyst stage, we were down to just four beautiful embryos. I transferred two and froze the remaining two embryos. It was scary to go from nineteen embryos to four, but I'm glad I waited because it worked."

—LANA

GAMETE INTRAFALLOPIAN TRANSFER (GIFT) AND ZYGOTE INTRAFALLOPIAN TRANSFER (ZIFT)

Most ARTs consist of some form of IVF, but some clinics still offer GIFT (gamete intrafallopian transfer) and ZIFT (zygote intrafallopian transfer). GIFT and ZIFT are somewhat simpler and less stressful than traditional IVF, although both require a normally functioning fallopian tube and laparoscopic surgery. While GIFT and ZIFT both achieve respectable pregnancy rates, generally more eggs or fertilized embryos are transferred earlier in their development to achieve these results. Then you're faced with higher rates of ectopic and multiple pregnancies, often with three or more fetuses at a time. These serious risks, coupled with the slightly higher costs ($15,000 to $20,000), make IVF usually a more cost-effective choice.

EGG FREEZING

Sperm and embryos are relatively easy to freeze, but embryologists have had very limited success in freezing eggs. While still not widely available (fewer than 250 babies have been born worldwide from egg freezing), this technology is improving. If ultimately successful, women will be able to extend their fertility by banking their eggs for later use.

A handful of companies advertise they can freeze and store your eggs now for about $13,000 for the initial egg retrieval and freezing technologies, plus about $500 a year for storage. Is this a good deal? Probably not, unless you are undergoing chemotherapy and have no other choices, or if you can participate in a clinical trial where treatment is free.

Egg freezing is still experimental. We simply know too little about egg freezing right now, including how long eggs can be frozen, how they are affected once they thaw, and what the actual pregnancy rates are. Forgive the bad cliché, but don't put all your eggs in this basket.

CYTOPLASMIC TRANSFER

This is where cytoplasm—the jellylike soup that holds a cell's contents from a healthy donor egg—is implanted into a patient's weaker egg to help it survive. The purpose is to produce an embryo with the genetic make-up of both parents, providing an alternative to egg donation. Cytoplasmic transfer is considered a highly experimental and controversial technique, with serious ethical concerns. Only a few clinics worldwide offer this technology (it is banned in the United States). Since it is highly experimental, there is little information about the cost. Expect to pay at least $20,000 to $40,000, not including the costs of traveling to one of the few clinics that offer it. Even less is known about the outcomes, since only about thirty children worldwide have been born as the result of this procedure. All of these children are still babies, so we don't yet know if there are future costs of this genetic manipulation.

Ongoing Costs: Frozen Embryos

Once your infertility treatments are complete, costs can still continue. If you have leftover embryos from ARTs, you need to consider the expenses of freezing and storing them through cyropreservation. These costs differ from clinic to clinic. First, there is the initial cost of freezing, which can be somewhere between $500 and $2,000. Then there are the annual storage fees, which range from $500 to $2,000 per year.

If you're not sure what to do with your cryopreserved embryos, this can add up to years of storage fees. But they can come in handy, since they can be used for additional frozen-cycle IVF attempts or frozen embryo transfer (FET) cycles. Because FET cycles do not involve the high costs of ovulation induction and egg retrieval, they cost considerably less, starting at about $1,000 to $3,000 plus any necessary medications per frozen embryo transfer. The good news is that research now shows IVF attempts with frozen embryos are at least as successful as fresh. So it's definitely worth keeping those cryopreserved embryos around if you think there is any chance you might want to try for another baby.

Occasionally, clinics will suggest you not freeze your embryos. They might insist you don't have anything worth freezing. Each clinic is different. Ask about your clinic's freezing criteria and how they determine whether or not to freeze an embryo. This is a tough call because it does cost to freeze embryos, and you don't want to waste your money if the odds aren't in your favor. But if there is any chance that these embryos might work, an FET is a whole lot cheaper than a fresh IVF cycle.

The clinic's reasons for discouraging you from cryopreserving might not be completely altruistic. Some clinics are running out of room to keep these frozen embryos on ice, so they look for opportunities to reduce the newcomers. Also, by not freezing your embryos, you are more likely to return to the clinic for a more expensive fresh cycle and not the cheaper frozen one. When making this decision, be a smart consumer and understand all your options. In the end, it's your money and your decision. If you want to freeze your leftover embryos, it's your call no matter what anyone else says.

In order to save yourself money and frustration later, consider how your embryos will be frozen and stored. Once they are thawed, you must use them or lose them. In other words, you must transfer them all to your uterus since embryos cannot be refrozen. To make the most of your frozen embryos, it helps to freeze them in smaller batches (maybe two or three to a straw) instead of freezing them all together. This way, you only need to freeze the ones you plan to transfer in that cycle. Of course, this involves more effort on the part of your clinic, not to mention your additional storage straws will take up slightly more room in their cryopreservation tank, but it's your right to make the most of your money.

Even families who do not wish to have more children are reluctant to forgo their embryos when the time comes. Research is improving each year and there have been new advances in developing personalized stem cell lines. It's easy to imagine a time when these embryos may one day benefit your family. You will ultimately have to decide if it is worth keeping these embryos indefinitely. Other choices include letting them just thaw, donating them to another infertile couple, or possibly letting them be used in research. The longer you put off making a decision about those embryos, the more money it's going to cost.

What's Right for You?

You will make decisions about your fertility treatment based on a variety of factors, including financial, psychological, and religious. With your partner, if applicable, sit down with the Fertility Action Plan in the appendix and discuss your options and which you may or may not be willing to consider and why.

Five Things You Can Do Right Now

1. Evaluate which additional testing may be right for you.
2. Consider if you meet the criteria for successful IVF.
3. Learn more about the specific procedure you are choosing so you can give yourself the best chance for success.
4. Think outside the box and explore other options for family building, such as egg or embryo donation.
5. If third-party assistance will be needed, find support now to prepare yourself emotionally.

CHAPTER 7

It's Easy to Get Lost:
Navigate the Insurance Maze

"I actually have good infertility insurance coverage; it covers three lifetime IVF attempts. This coverage let me choose the alternative with the least medical risk: single-embryo transfers. If I had to pay for it myself, I might have pushed for transferring two. My clinic would not allow me to transfer three unless I had multiple failed prior attempts. The 'three tries' limit also encouraged me to cancel my cycles that were not turning out well, prior to the egg retrieval procedure.

"For me, three attempts is sufficient coverage. If IVF is going to work for me, it probably will within that many attempts. And many people don't have the emotional energy to go through more than two attempts anyway. However this last cycle turns out, I'll know I did everything I could."

—KIM

IS YOUR INSURANCE COMPANY EVIL? Does it exist solely to keep you from getting pregnant? No, not really. It just seems that way sometimes. Most of us struggle to understand what our health insurance policy covers. Unfair denials, late payments, voice mail hell, and hopeless confusion seem to be the norm. Trying to get your insurance company to pony up the big bucks for infertility seems like an exercise in futility. But sometimes, it works. We'll teach you how.

Does Your Insurance Company Have It In for You?

Winston Churchill once described the former Soviet Union as "a riddle wrapped in a mystery inside an enigma." The same is true for understanding infertility treatment coverage in health insurance. Insurers now offer coverage for the various stages of infertility treatment—from examinations and tests to procedures and medications. Regardless of where your insurance policy falls, you need to dig it out, find a microscope for all that fine print, and settle in for some important, if not scintillating, reading.

It's time to get down to business. You need to learn the nuts and bolts of your health care plan. That's the key to success, says Rhonda Orin, attorney and author of *Making Them Pay: How to Get the Most from Health Insurance and Managed Care*.

"The truth is, it can be tough to get your insurance company to pay for infertility treatment," says Orin. "Infertility treatment is a gray area—it's potentially very expensive, and they are going to try to avoid paying if they can, even if it's covered. You have to know your policy. Know it word for word. Really study it. Be your own best advocate."

A LITTLE FREE ASSISTANCE

One of the pharmaceutical companies that wants to promote their infertility medications to potential patients offers a free, educational resource for people struggling with infertility. By calling Fertility Lifelines at 1-800-LETS-TRY or by visiting their website at www.fertilitylifelines.com, you can talk to a trained benefits specialist or a fertility nurse. Provided by EMD Serono, this service might be able to help you save a little time in understanding your health benefits and any infertility coverage you might have, but always remember their ultimate goal is to push their meds.

Where Do I Start?

Do not set foot in a stirrup until you figure out what all that gobbledygook means in the health insurance folder you shoved in a drawer somewhere. Know what your policy covers *before* you see a health care provider. A common mistake people make is they expect their health care providers to let them know what's covered.

"Trust me: your health care provider does not know what is covered!" explains Toni Siragusa, a certified financial planner. "[Your provider] outlines a plan of treatment for you, then the billing department calls or bills your insurer for the treatment they have provided to you. Your health care provider does not always take the time to confirm what is covered." Additionally, they can make the mistake in thinking that you have the same insurance as other patients, but your contract may be different, even if it is the same insurance company. You need to review this information yourself—the type of contract you have dictates your coverage, what kind of health care provider you see, the kinds of tests you undergo, the sequence of the testing, and what treatments will be covered (and at what rate).

First, find and read your policy. Go ahead—even if you think you already know what it says. If you are enrolled in an employer-sponsored health plan, you should have received what is called a Summary Plan Description when you first signed up. If you have only the one- or two-page summary of benefits, you don't have everything you need. (If only it were that easy!) Although this document may summarize your coverage in language that's easy to understand, it is not the legal document that will be used if your dispute with your health plan ends up in court. For a complete description of your plan's benefits, contact your employer's human resources department for a copy of what is known as the "Evidence of Coverage" or "Certificate of Insurance."

If you bought your own health plan, you should have received the Evidence of Coverage when you bought the policy. If you are not sure if you have the most recent copy, check with your health plan's customer service department or your insurance agent.

Don't go get the policy that's been moldering in the back of your filing cabinet. They change at least annually. Every so often, the carrier throws in addendums that can fundamentally alter your plan. You know how your company sends you letters letting you know when there's a policy change? You're actually supposed to read those. Who knew? Get the newest booklet from your HR department. Don't even try to use an old copy. You can check to see if the most recent one is available online, but you need a hard copy as well.

Even understanding the sections of your policy is tricky, Orin explains. Look for the section titled "Benefits." It is usually broken into five parts:

- Medical/Surgery
- Prescription Drugs

- Extended Care
- Emergency Care
- Mental Health

The most recent benefits that have either increased or decreased are listed in an addendum in the front of the booklet. You'll need to review both your medical and prescription coverage.

What to Look For
- What is the definition of "infertility" specified in the contract?
- What infertility coverage is listed—from no coverage to full coverage?
- What procedures or procedure codes require preauthorization?
- Are there restrictions on the type of health care provider who can perform fertility services?
- What tests need to be done before you can be diagnosed with infertility?
- Do you need a referral to see a fertility specialist?
- What limits, if any, apply to your coverage—in terms of treatment cycles, procedures, months in therapy, et cetera?
- Is there drug coverage?
- Are infertility drugs covered under the pharmacy benefit or medical benefit?
- Do you need to go to a specific pharmacy to fill your prescriptions?
- Are there specific pharmacy restrictions?

Use the "Evaluating Your Insurance Coverage" chart in the appendix to organize your insurance benefits.

Types of Plans

Insurance plans come in all shapes and sizes, and no two are alike. The type of plan you have will have a huge bearing on your overall coverage. *Indemnity insurance* (also called fee-for-service) pays for most of your major medical treatments, but it usually doesn't pay for preventive care or non-life-threatening problems, like infertility. And indemnity insurance does not cover the total cost of anything. You are required to pay a percentage of the billed amount. Since you are paying such a large amount of your health care out-of-pocket, you are able to see any doctor or hospital you want with this type of plan.

A *preferred provider organization (PPO)* covers many of your health care needs for a small per-visit fee if you choose from the list of "preferred providers." If you choose to see a doctor who is "out of network," you will be responsible for a greater part of the bill. Because of the nature of the field, most fertility specialists are not a part of any preferred provider networks. However, if you find one that is, you will save quite a bit of cash by staying "in network."

A *health maintenance organization (HMO)* pays for most of your health care, including preventive care, for a small copayment per visit. With an HMO, there are no claim forms, but you can use only doctors affiliated with your plans. Coverage is limited only to specialty services authorized by your primary care physician with a written referral. Unless you are affiliated with a large HMO like Kaiser Permanente of California, it is unlikely that the treatment of infertility would fall into this. Even if it does, you will be required to pay more of the treatment costs than just your copay.

Types of Benefits

The coverage problem results from the way health insurance coverage defines "medical necessity." Most health insurance policies will reimburse tests and procedures they consider medically necessary to diagnose and treat an individual for sickness, illness, or disease. For example, most health insurance companies consider diabetes or hypertension serious diseases and fully expect to reimburse the costs for the diagnosis and treatment of these conditions. Unfortunately, not everyone sees infertility as a disease.

Infertility health insurance coverage varies widely across the United States, and insurance carriers view infertility treatment as elective or not medically necessary. A few health plans offer no infertility benefits, many offer diagnostic infertility benefits and limited treatment benefits, some offer specific dollar limits for both diagnosis and treatment, and only a few plans offer unlimited infertility diagnosis and treatment benefits.

DIFFERENT LEVELS OF INFERTILITY COVERAGE

No infertility benefit. This total lack of infertility coverage is uncommon. You can still usually get diagnostic testing done, especially if you have PCOS, endometriosis, or other health problems that affect more than just fertility.

Diagnostic testing only. This is the most common type of benefit and covers procedures necessary to diagnose the causes of infertility, such as ultrasound, HSG, hormone levels, and semen analysis. It also covers diagnostic surgeries such as hysteroscopy and laparoscopy.

Diagnostic testing and limited treatment. Benefits include diagnostic testing and treatment limited to ovulation induction and/or artificial insemination. Drug benefits may include clomiphene citrate and, less commonly, the injectable medications.

All treatments are covered. This is the rarest but most generous policy, though it can change year to year. Coverage includes IVF treatment and injectable medications. There is often a limit on the amount covered or the number of IVF attempts allowed.

What Doesn't It Say?

Read your contract to determine if there is a specific exclusion for infertility. Generally speaking, if the contract does not have exclusion for infertility, the insurance company must pay benefits. But if there is an exclusion, carefully read what it excludes. Does it exclude treatments only, or does it also exclude diagnosis?

For example, a woman had a laparoscopy because of pelvic pain. The insurance carrier denied the claim, stating it was for the treatment of infertility. By taking the claim through the grievance process, eventually the insurance carrier paid because it wasn't done for infertility, but for pelvic pain. Since the procedure was diagnostic, the insurance carrier determined it was required to make the payment.

If your policy does not have an exclusion for infertility treatment, it may refuse coverage only for specific situations. For example, some policies will exclude infertility treatment for patients who have undergone a sterilization procedure (tubal ligation or vasectomy) or who are undergoing natural menopause.

WHO IS ELIGIBLE FOR FERTILITY INSURANCE?

Although it varies from insurer to insurer, there are normally certain qualifications that you have to meet before being approved for fertility insurance by your insurance plan. For example, most often you will need to:

- Be under the age of 40
- Have struggled with infertility for a specific time (ranging from one to five years)
- Be a policyholder for at least one year

Also, couples that do not have insurance coverage and are currently undergoing infertility treatment will most likely not be approved for fertility coverage.

Be the First to Find Out

It's tempting to let someone else do the detective work and decipher what your insurance company pays. That's what the front office at the fertility clinic is there for, right? Even some drug companies have insurance advocates who will offer to do this for you for free. Accept all the help you can get, but do your own homework.

Just because the scuttlebutt around the water cooler suggests absolutely nothing infertility-related is covered in your company health plan doesn't mean it's true. Often, people who've experienced dissatisfaction in trying to obtain insurance coverage will freely dispense misinformation to others. They might be right, but they may have missed something (or a lot of somethings). Even for people who work at the same company, your health insurance policies might be drastically different. Regardless, your situation is different and your outcomes may be different as well. Never assume that just because a friend's or colleague's fertility treatment was or wasn't covered, your experience will be the same.

Never trust the doctor's office to find out if you are covered. They generally check for individual procedures as they arise and not the totality of coverage. Women have made decisions about their treatment based on what somebody in the clinic's office thought she understood—and it was wrong! Plus, while the clinics want you to get treatment, the clinic makes more money and gets paid faster if you pay yourself. Keep in mind that clinics are not going to rock the boat with insurance companies they must maintain long-term relationships with.

As impatient as you are to get things started, you must get a commitment for coverage prior to seeing a fertility specialist. This is called preauthorization or predetermination. You must write a letter requesting preauthorization to your insurance company.

Get It in Writing

"I stood in the driveway with my mouth open, looking at the bill from my doctor. It was wrong. It had to be. I called the insurance company so my testing and blood work would be covered before I had it done. I talked to the person on the phone and had her name and everything. But it didn't matter. When the clinic filed the claim, the insurance company said it wasn't covered and refused to pay the $3,500 bill. I had to pay every penny of it."
—Pauline

"The over-the-phone approval doesn't mean all that much," explains Rhonda Orin. "Don't bother making the call. It is a waste of your time. And it will just make you crazy having to deal with them." After all, it sounds easier to make a call than to write a letter, but it's not. You know the drill. First, you're on hold, then you're punching in random numbers, then you get a voice mail, and so on. Any time the insurance guys say they are going to pay for something, you want it in writing and on their letterhead. Sample precertification letters are included in the appendix.

Why? Because the insurance company can deny a claim once the bill is turned in, even if you called and got approval first. We know it's not fair, but this is why you have to do this right. Although it can still happen, it is much more difficult for them to deny a claim if you have it in black and white that they'll pay.

Don't Risk It!
Do not proceed with treatment until you have the insurer's precertification letter in your hand! It's better to postpone an appointment than to go in with no information or the wrong information about your coverage.

This is important: you must send all letters to the insurance company via certified mail. All correspondence to the insurance company needs to be sent this way. Although you can never be sure that someone actually read your letter, it does provide some proof of your communication. And no, email is not mail and does not count, and neither does a fax. Use a certified letter because it gives you a mailing receipt from the US Postal Service. Plus, for less than $5, a record of delivery is maintained at the addressee's post office for six months, you can follow the letter online, and if you want, you can even request a copy of the signature record. In other words, they can't say they never got your letter. You've got proof they did. And ignoring your request for a hearing, for example, can land them in deep trouble.

But here's the sneaky part: the postal service won't deliver certified letters to post office boxes. And most insurance companies guard their mailing addresses carefully and give out addresses only with post office boxes. Even the letterhead sent to their customers rarely offers the real address. The mailing address for appeals is listed at the very end of your benefits book. Use this address, as it is the official address for appeals for the company—

To Find the Insurance Commission in Your State
Contact the National Association of Insurance Commissioners at www.naic.org or 816-842-3600.

the beginning of the process. You can also go online and use the corporate HQ. You may want to send a certified letter to *both* addresses.

Crack the Codes

There are two kinds of codes in your medical records: a diagnostic code and a procedural code. The diagnostic codes are known as ICD-9 codes and explain the diagnosis or what is causing your inability to become pregnant. The procedural codes are CPT codes for the treatment provided. Many insurance plans will cover basic diagnostics, even if they don't pay for treatments.

Anything officially infertility related will not be covered by most insurance. On the other hand, reproductive problems impacting your general health, such as ovulation problems, PCOS, and endometriosis, just might be covered. A few digits can make the difference as to whether or not you're covered! For example, if your doctor's office bills you for infertility instead of endometriosis, you might not be covered. Or the wrong code might be typed in accidentally, and if you don't watch your bills carefully, you won't notice it or understand why the claim was denied. The appendix includes common diagnostic and billing codes you might need to become familiar with. Your doctor cannot deliberately file an incorrect code—it's insurance fraud. In other words, if it really is an infertility treatment, the office can't file it as something else.

Comparison Shopping

Compare your insurance policy against your partner's policy. If their insurance is more comprehensive, it may be better to switch policies or add a secondary policy. If you aren't sure what's covered in a policy you are considering, call the company's 800 number. If you do call, call more than once at different times of the day to speak to different customer service representatives.

If you are married or have partner benefits with both employers, talk to both human resources departments about how to arrange coordination of benefits between you and your partner. Find out if there are any differences in coverage between the primary holder and dependents.

WHAT TO CONSIDER WHEN COMPARING POLICIES

- Are drug benefits listed separately from infertility treatment benefits?

- Does your policy cover complementary treatments, such as massage therapy and acupuncture?

- Are there any other factors you need to consider (doctor limitations, other physical ailments, et cetera)?

- Are mental health benefits covered? Many individuals and couples find they need extra help with the stress and find outpatient therapy visits helpful.

- What is the level of maternity and prenatal care coverage, considering some ART pregnancies are considered high-risk?

- What are the preexisting conditions, since rules differ widely by policy?

You may also have an opportunity to comparison shop within your own company. While some companies will let you change at any time, many limit insurance switches to a specific time period called open enrollment. Open enrollment is typically scheduled toward the end of the calendar year. Find out when yours is by calling your HR department.

Other sources for health insurance may be a better fit. Check with any professional organizations you belong to or are eligible to join. Those groups—which represent a spectrum of professionals from lawyers and real-

DURING OPEN ENROLLMENT, YOU CAN

- Change to a different medical plan

- Opt out of medical, dental, and/or vision coverage or cancel a previous opt-out request

- Enroll eligible family members in your health plan

- Cancel coverage for a currently enrolled family member

- Enroll or reenroll in the Health Care Reimbursement Account

tors and even performers, writers, and photographers, to some freelancers—may be able to meet your needs.

Secondary Insurance

Since many people have access to medical insurance from more than one plan (such as two employed spouses covered under group health insurance plans), insurance companies do not want the insured to profit through their health insurance. To prevent double recovery, most health insurance plans have provisions that determine how primary versus secondary coverage will be determined.

Primary coverage is provided through the plan of which they are a member (such as the spouses both covered through their respective employment; the primary coverage is provided under the plan held by the employer of each spouse) or the plan under which the member has been a participant for the longest time period.

Secondary coverage is usually a result of being covered as a dependent under someone else's health insurance plan or buying a second plan on your own and provides reimbursement for medical expenses *after* exhaustion of coverage through the primary plan. What are the benefits of secondary insurance? Secondary insurance covers a portion of what your primary insurance doesn't cover. That might mean copays for doctor visits and medications to deductibles for hospitalization to formula. They may also cover services such as treatments and private duty nursing. If you can swing it, many believe it is well worth the hassle and expense.

> *"When I decided to go out of state for my infertility treatments, I bought another individual policy from a reputable insurance company on top of my existing HMO. For about $200 a month, I got multiple cycles with an 80 percent reimbursement. However, I did have to fight hard for this, but it worked out in the end."*
>
> —Tess

The Devil Is in the Details: Referrals and Authorizations

Depending on your insurance plan, a referral from your PCP, primary care physician or "gatekeeper" physician, is sometimes necessary for your first fertility specialist visit. In some cases a gynecologist is considered your PCP; other times, you might have to see a family practitioner or internist before you can visit a fertility specialist. Check the rules with your insurance plan to ensure that you fill out all the paperwork correctly. A verbal or professional referral is not the same as a formal referral for insurance purposes. It doesn't count as a formal referral when your gynecologist mentions you should see a fertility specialist. Most major plans have a phone number listed on the insurance card you can call to get information and authorization.

Since it may take up to several weeks with some insurance companies to authorize your treatment, plan accordingly. If you don't have a referral or an authorization, your insurance will not reimburse your visit and you will ultimately be responsible for the cost.

If you are covered by a health maintenance organization (HMO), you must use its network of providers. While states require HMOs to have adequate networks of qualified providers, not all HMOs do. If there are not such providers located near you, you can ask the state to intervene or the HMO to make an exception for you. If you have a point of service (POS) plan, where you have the option of going out of network, you will be responsible for the deductibles and copayments. And the costs for going out of network are going to be much higher as well.

Preexisting Conditions

If you or your partner changes jobs and your insurance changes, what happens if you are in the middle of making choices about infertility treatment? The easy answer: it depends. Generally, the rules about preexisting conditions are located in the back of the benefits booklet. If your primary diagnosis is endometriosis, for example, then your new insurance may refuse to provide treatment for endometriosis for a predetermined period of time, generally three to six months. Again, find out exactly what is covered—and when—by getting it in writing.

Those who must pay out of pocket for infertility treatments do not generally have to wait for the preexisting clause. If your insurance will be picking up some of the tab, some companies will put limitations on coverage if you have been through some infertility treatment already. For example, if your previous insurance covered two IVF cycles, and your new policy provides a lifetime maximum of four cycles, the new company may count those previous two cycles against you and allow only two more. Don't intentionally provide wrong information or leave out important details. You can get busted for insurance fraud.

The insurance industry has this sneaky little thing called the MIB, the Medical Information Bureau. Operating like a medical version of your credit report, there is a record on you if you have applied for life, health, or disability insurance in the last seven years. Insurance companies can find out if you're a smoker, are routinely in car accidents, or have other health problems. In other words, if you deny seeking infertility treatment and the new insurance company finds out you did, it can ask you to return the amount it's spent on you and refuse further infertility treatment. To get a copy of your free MIB report, call the toll-free number at 866-692-6901 or go to www.MIB.com.

But don't be too willing to elaborate on your entire past medical history to just anyone. Verify what they need, why they need it, and where they are getting their information. Understand your rights and responsibilities as a patient. Know if what they are asking violates HIPAA (the Health Insurance Portability and Privacy Act), which ensures the security and privacy of everyone's personal health data. For information about HIPAA, contact www.hhs.gov/ocr/hipaa/.

Lifetime Maximums

"I have $20,000 lifetime max. I started getting denials in the mail from my insurance company, stating I was maxed out after just one cycle! I called and requested a detailed list of each service because I had a hunch my fertility specialist billed wrong. About two weeks later, I received a letter from the insurance company that they had audited the fertility specialist's charges and found I still had over $14,000 in coverage available! My fertility specialist was billing

things like labs and ultrasounds as infertility when the retrieval and transfer costs are the only fees that count toward my lifetime maximum!"

—LEAH

Don't get too excited about having infertility coverage until you find out what your lifetime maximum is. Here's the bummer. Lifetime maximums often cap at $5,000 to $15,000. But you can save money on the lifetime max clause in some cases. For example, if you go to your gynecologist for an annual exam and get your hormones checked, it may be covered under your wellness care and not counted toward your lifetime infertility maximum.

When is the maximum not the maximum? Pay close attention to the details here. When your insurance limits you to a lifetime maximum of infertility treatment dollars, do they mean the lifetime of your coverage with that company under this specific contract, or do they mean your literal, actual lifetime? The answer, once again, is it depends on the contract. Lifetime max can mean the lifetime maximum for that insurance policy in a nonmandated state (we will discuss the differences between mandated and nonmandated states later on in this chapter). So, for example, should you have a lifetime max with a self-insured plan and max out, if you select another policy, you may be able to start over. In New Jersey, and some other mandated states, the lifetime max is the lifetime of your treatment, and it would not start over. (See page 122 for a discussion of mandates.)

Cycle Limits

Even knowing how many IVF cycles your insurance covers may not be as cut and dried as you thought. Find out how an IVF cycle is defined. For some, it is defined as a cycle that results in an embryo transfer. If something goes wrong and the eggs don't fertilize, or other glitches that prohibit transfer occur, then that cycle doesn't count toward your maximum. You may have more chances than you thought.

But some insurance companies view any attempt (even a cycle that doesn't make it to embryo transfer) as a full cycle. This is your responsibility to track. For example, Gayle assumed her doctor's office was appropriately managing all of the insurance paperwork for her. Unfortunately, her fertility clinic submitted the bill for a canceled cycle directly to her insurance company. She was livid when she found she wasted her last insurance-covered cycle on a $2,000 canceled attempt. It would have been smarter to pay for that cycle out of pocket and have her insurance company foot the bill for a subsequent $15,000 cycle. Now she doesn't have the money to try again and there is nothing she can do about this billing mistake. Lesson learned: Never hand over responsibility for understanding your coverage to your clinic.

Contracted Rates

Insurance companies have predetermined contracted rates that are far below the retail cost of the doctor bills. The rates vary, but insurance companies pay considerably less than the actual billed amount. In some cases, doctor visits are reimbursed at 50 percent below normal retail rates, or the fee you would be charged if you paid directly.

If you do not have insurance, or are "underinsured," you do not have access to these contracted rates. So if you need medical care, you are responsible to pay for the complete billed amount. In other words, if you're covered for ultrasounds by your insurance, the insurance company will probably pay the negotiated rate of about $75. If you don't have insurance, you're stuck with the full $300 bill for the same procedure.

What's a State Mandate?

As of this writing, fifteen states have passed legislation requiring insurers to cover infertility treatments. Each state law is different and can be divided into two groups: those that mandate to cover and those that mandate to offer. Most states have no such laws, and there is no federal law requiring that insurance plans cover infertility services. Mandated benefits vary by state, and each state has its own rules, loopholes, and exclusions. A complete list of state mandates is available in appendix 11 and updated frequently on our web page.

MANDATE TO COVER

A mandate to cover generally means health insurance companies must provide infertility diagnosis and treatment for all policyholders. Eleven states have mandates that coverage be provided; however, these mandates vary. Some of them mandate coverage be provided only by certain forms of health insurance, such as HMOs, and many direct certain medical conditions be met before coverage is provided. Some specifically mandate coverage for assisted reproductive technologies (ART), while others specifically limit or exclude it.

In some states, such as Massachusetts, the law mandates the couple has to try to conceive naturally for a year before the insurance can cover any fertility treatments. This is fine for most couples, but not for those over forty who do not have time to wait one year. And if you get pregnant during this year and miscarry, your one-year wait time starts all over again.

STATES THAT HAVE MANDATED HEALTH INSURANCE PLANS INCLUDING COVERAGE OF ALL OR SOME ASPECTS OF INFERTILITY SERVICES

- Arkansas
- Connecticut
- Hawaii
- Illinois
- Maryland
- Massachusetts
- Montana
- New Jersey
- New York
- Ohio
- Rhode Island
- West Virginia

MANDATE TO OFFER

Some states have a mandate-to-offer law. A mandate-to-offer requirement means there is a law requiring health insurance companies to at least offer employers policies that cover infertility diagnosis and treatment. However, laws do not require employers to purchase such policies, so employers do not have to provide infertility coverage as a standard part of their plans. California and Texas both require companies to make available policies that cover infertility treatment.

Why Mandates Are Not a Done Deal

"I work for a New Jersey company. As a result, I thought in vitro fertilization would be covered. The company headquarters is in New Jersey and the plan is administered in New Jersey. I also live in New Jersey. But they wrote the plan out of their New York office. As a result, I'm not entitled to IVF! I am covered under the New Jersey state law only if the insurance policy is issued in New Jersey."

—SALLY

Even if you live in a state with mandated coverage, you may not have full benefits. Certain companies, such as those with fewer than fifty employees, are exempt from state regulation of health insurance. Under the Employment Retirement Security Act of 1974 (ERISA), companies with self-funded health plans are exempt from state health insurance laws of any kind, including infertility mandates.

What's the difference between self-insured versus fully insured? Large companies and unions tend to self-insure their benefits. Although they may use an Aetna or Blue Cross to administer their benefits, process their claims, and answer phone calls, it's the employer who pays the claims. Your employer assumes the risk of all the costs.

The larger the company, the more likely they are to be self-insured. In some states, more than 50 percent of employees work for employers exempted under ERISA. Fortunately, self-insured employers sometimes do choose to follow the state's policy lead and provide infertility coverage to their employees.

Options in Mandated States

What if you live in a mandated state, but your employer has a loophole making it exempt? Some enterprising folks have started their own companies, and as boss and employee, bought insurance coverage. Of course, you choose a plan that excludes nothing from the coverage. If you have a hobby or interest, it costs about $100 to get a business license, depending on the town you operate your business in. Want to get started selling your writing, marketing your scrapbook services, or other goods? You don't have to show a profit. Check with your local chamber of commerce to locate potential insurance plans.

The catch is the address can't be a post office box, but any other address will work. UPS stores work as well, since they have a street address. If you have a sole proprietorship, there is no tax ID necessary, and a simple schedule C tax form will suffice. However, this is still going to be pricey, usually over $1,000 per month.

States Without Mandates

The remaining thirty-six states do not have laws requiring the provision or offer of infertility coverage. There are infertility advocacy organizations actively campaigning for adoption of additional state infertility insurance mandates. Currently, campaigns to enact such mandates are particularly active in Florida, Maine, and Pennsylvania. There also are ongoing efforts to strengthen the existing mandates in Massachusetts and Texas.

Federal Employees

Although fertility testing and diagnostics are usually covered, there is no federal law requiring coverage for infertility treatments. As a result, federal employees must pay for all infertility treatment expenses out of pocket, even if they live in a mandated state. Besides helping federal employees, a federal infertility insurance mandate, a long-term goal of the infertility community, would cover all employers and make coverage consistent across states.

The US Military and Fertility Treatment

Trying to understand military health insurance makes deconstructing traditional policies look easy. TRICARE is the health insurance program for active-duty and retired members of the uniformed services, their families, and survivors. If you or your partner are in the military, gaining access to infertility coverage depends on a number of different factors, including where you're stationed, how long it takes for referrals to wind their way through the system in your area, and if the military member gets deployed in the middle of the process!

> *"My advice is to keep bugging them. If you talk to fifty different people, you'll get fifty different answers about what's covered. Some people I know got stuff paid for, while others didn't . . . keep trying until you find one person who will help you and get you what you need."*
>
> —AMY

Will TRICARE pay for infertility treatment? Not exactly. TRICARE covers only the diagnostic workup to identify the underlying cause of infertility. It will, however, cover treatment for the underlying cause. For example, most military bases will do vasectomy reversals for free, although there may be a waiting list.

Generally, TRICARE covers all of the blood work and all of the ultrasounds and monitoring. Some medications used in a cycle (i.e., estrogen, Provera) are covered under TRICARE, or you can get them free on base. Officially, injectable gonadotropins are not covered under the TRICARE pharmacy benefit if they are being prescribed for use in conjunction with an ART, including but not limited to IUI, IVF, or GIFT. So they will approve them for ovulation induction cycles with timed intercourse, but probably not for anything else. Still, some women get the claim filled. Results seem to be spotty and depend on a wide variety of factors, including the mood of the person processing your claim.

Getting started on infertility treatment while in the military isn't easy. First, make an appointment with your gynecologist or primary care physician. Schedule a yearly physical along with this appointment to get a Pap smear and an overall checkup. Then tell your doctor you want a referral to see a fertility specialist. You may have to really push for an outside referral. Keep coming back until you get a referral. Some women report being given eighteen months of clomiphene citrate and told to come back if they aren't pregnant when the prescription runs out. Don't accept more than four months of clomiphene citrate. It's a waste of your precious fertile time and money.

> *"It took forever to be taken seriously about not getting pregnant. I had to go to my primary care provider three times in one month to complain about various female problems. Finally, she got tired of seeing me and she referred me on."*
>
> —SUE

The care you receive may depend on how old you are; the younger you are, the longer they make you wait. If you're over thirty, usually they tell you to have unprotected sex for six months first. If you have documentation (charting for six months; twelve months if you're younger), you should be able to gain access faster.

In terms of third-party reproduction, TRICARE has changed its policy very recently and will no longer pay for anything related to a surrogacy pregnancy. TRICARE has even begun to deny maternity benefits for military wives serving as surrogates while their husbands are deployed.

ON-BASE CARE

TRICARE does not cover IVF, but there are several military facilities that offer ART programs. Generally, by using military physicians, patients are charged for only laboratory services. Programs and fees vary, but IVF costs are usually around $5,000 to $8,000.

MILITARY HOSPITALS WITH IVF PROGRAMS

Balboa Naval Hospital, San Diego
Tripler Army Medical Center, Hawaii
Walter Reed, Washington, DC
Wilford Hall Medical Center, Lackland AFB, Texas
Madigan Army Medical Center, Washington state

Their success rates are published with the CDC reports, but these clinics often cap a woman's age at forty. In addition, unlike most private clinics, cycles are usually batched four times yearly, meaning you can cycle only during those periods. In addition, there may be other requirements or limitations you wouldn't find at a clinic off-base. For example, for most military clinics, no donor eggs are allowed, the woman may not be obese, and the couple must not be receiving marital counseling.

IVF at these military facilities will be done only after you have been given a referral from your primary care physician. And after getting a referral, it can take from six months to a year for a consultation, and it can take a year or longer to get into a program. A number of tests must be completed before admission to the program, but they cannot be more than a year old. Expect a waiting list, but these treatment centers are good options if you have time to wait and you are persistent.

Persistence, persistence, persistence. It is easy to get lost in the system. If you want to get anywhere with infertility treatment as a member of the military, be prepared to fight every inch of the way. It may go smoothly, and you may not need to, but you must be your own advocate.

OFF-BASE CARE

It's a crapshoot here. No one really knows what TRICARE will pay for if you go to a fertility clinic, but don't expect much. Some clinics offer a discount payment plan for military families seeking IVF. It doesn't hurt to ask. If your clinic doesn't publicize a military discount, ask if they would consider giving one.

Some clinics also provide free sperm storage for those members of the active military who are going into combat. This service protects the ability of servicemen to become fathers after their return from duty should they lose it as a result of injury. Ask your local clinic if it would be willing to match these offers.

Fertility Insurance

"After my last IVF cycle, I had a bad case of ovarian hyper-stimulation. I was in the hospital for four days because of the severe vomiting and bloating. I couldn't get in and out of bed independently, and had difficulty moving around. My vomiting was so violent that I cracked one of my ribs. Needless to say, I

missed two weeks of work, which did not go over well with my
boss, since I had taken so much time off to do the cycle. I didn't have
any sick time left, and between the hospital and missed work, it cost
an extra couple thousand we weren't planning on."

—LEANN

While you can't buy a health insurance policy just for infertility treatment, you can buy infertility insurance that protects you from the financial risks of complications from a procedure. For example, in Leann's case, such insurance would have provided short-term disability and medical costs for any complications resulting from infertility treatments. It can also provide long-term disability protection should you be unable to work and suffer a loss of income following complications from a procedure. In a worst-case scenario, you can also buy life insurance in case an infertility procedure kills you, but you should have life insurance anyway.

Fertility insurance is usually mandatory for collaborative cycles like egg donation. It protects the donors from unforeseen and costly medical complications from donating. Surrogates are always provided with such insurance, and it is the responsibility of the recipient to provide.

Maternity Coverage

Once you get pregnant, your maternity insurance kicks in. Check your coverage now because once you get pregnant, it's considered a preexisting condition, so you usually cannot add on coverage for pregnancy and delivery. This is a huge expense you don't want to pay out of pocket. And if your baby is born with a problem or there are complications during childbirth, a hospital bill can be devastating.

Disability Insurance

"I signed up for disability insurance the week before I started my
first IVF. It was really cheap, and I started to panic about potential
dangers. When I became pregnant with the triplets, I delivered
early and I got paid $100 for each day I was in the hospital and so
did each of my babies. They were in NICU for two months! I know

in some states they exclude you if you have ever gone through infertility treatments or if the pregnancy resulted from infertility treatments, but it was the best spur-of-the-moment decision I ever made!"

—MATTIE

Some very generous companies automatically provide disability insurance. Most don't, but you can add it to your policy at work or purchase it on your own. Compare companies and their policies carefully, but you can usually get coverage for under $100 per month. If you get pregnant and end up on bed rest, you'll wish you had it. Plus, knowing your complete insurance benefits can affect your overall financial plan for having a baby.

Don't Forget About Your Clinic

All fertility clinics have at least one person, and sometimes two or three, on staff who deals only with insurance. Introduce yourself to these people. While you are ultimately responsible for understanding your insurance and managing claims, these people can be a great resource. After all, insurance is all they do, day in and day out. They should be up on all the issues, terminology, and codes in order for you to get the most out of your insurance. Medical insurance is a big issue for all of us. And odds are, they despise the insurance industry as much as you do. Like everything infertility-related, you can't expect to go in as a lone ranger. Pick their brains. Ask about insurance and infertility in general. Then inquire about your specific policy. What has their experience been in the past with your insurance company? What types of difficulties and barriers have they encountered? How can you best avoid additional problems? What are they going to do to ensure the maximum coverage? What do they suggest you do when speaking with your insurance company? It's best that you work with your clinic staff when dealing with insurance issues. With so many complexities and confusion surrounding insurance, two heads are way better than one.

Understanding your health insurance policy is a major accomplishment! Lesser mortals have trembled at the thought. One caveat: Just because you have insurance doesn't mean they'll pay the right amount. Or pay in a timely manner. They may even refuse your legitimate claim. But none of these is insurmountable, either. This information should help you battle for the coverage you deserve.

Five Things You Can Do Right Now

1. Get the most up-to-date policy information from your health insurer.
2. Request preauthorization letters for medical coverage and prescription benefits from your carrier.
3. Find the date for open enrollment for your and your partner's insurance so you know the time frame for making changes.
4. Start organizing your insurance records right now. Keep receipts for all out-of-pocket expenses. Make a folder right now. You may have enough expenses for a tax deduction come tax time (see chapter 12, page 225).
5. Consider adding short-term and/or long-term disability insurance to your coverage.

CHAPTER 8

The Medicine Cabinet:
Track Down Affordable Fertility Drugs

"My fertility specialist said it was time to start injectables, which I'd been dreading. Clomid was miserable, but these seem so much worse. High cost? Time off work? You bet. He said the cost would start from $1,750 per cycle just for the medication, and I should expect it to rise to around $4,000 per cycle, with ultrasounds and all that junk included. Also, he said I would need to be monitored, so I'd have to come in three or four days early in the morning to have ultrasounds and blood tests. So, I need to work next year in order to pay for all this, yet I can't really hold down a job if I have to miss that much work."

—CHLOE

ONE FERTILITY MEDICATION HAS SIDE effects that exactly mimic those of early pregnancy—tender breasts, nausea, uterine cramping—but also those of an impending period—bloating, depression, and insatiable cravings for carbohydrates. But wait! There's more! At no extra charge, we'll throw in wild mood swings. Now, how much would you pay? Forty dollars a vial? And that's just one of the infertility medications you'll need.

It's bad enough you have to inject hormones in your stomach, but since they represent 20 percent to 30 percent of the total expense of fertility care, we'll help you find the cheapest and safest medications. The constipation? You're on your own.

Drugs eat up a considerable portion of your expenses for IUI, IVF, and other fertility treatments. Depending on your age, ovarian response, diagnosis, and other factors, the cost of fertility meds varies greatly. While you have to take them, you can learn to save money and protect yourself at the same time.

Getting Started

Once you learn all the fertility terms, you've got to figure out the meds. For different types of procedures, different types and amounts of medications will be used. What you will need varies from woman to woman, and even clinic to clinic, but there are some standard protocols, so you can begin planning and knowing what to expect. One way to look at your potential prescription price tag is to get a ballpark figure of what most fertility specialists use. While drinking alcohol isn't recommended for women in fertility treatments, you might want to budget a glass or two for your partner.

No matter where you are in the process, one thing you can do right now is start taking prenatal vitamins. Go with the generic, which are less than $5 for one hundred. The most important ingredient in these is folic acid (folate), which may reduce the risk of certain birth defects such as spina bifida and other neural tube defects. Any prenatal vitamin with folic acid will do, even many children's vitamins. Most people have a prescription benefit card that will cover prenatal vitamins containing the recommended amount of folic acid. Don't waste your money on any so-called fertility-enhancing vitamins or any other supplements, some of which will set you back several hundred dollars a month. None of these has been scientifically proven to do any good, and sometimes they can even work against fertility medications.

Ovulation Induction

Ovulation induction, or stimulation, is the process of getting your ovaries to produce more eggs. After all, you need an egg to get pregnant. There are two main ways to do this, and they vary tremendously in cost. The first approach is to try with clomiphene citrate (more commonly known by the brand names Clomid or Serophene). This is the only time on the infertility roller coaster where you can get away with less than $100 for a medicated cycle. Clomiphene citrate is taken by mouth in the form of a little pill, is cheap, and helps a lot of women. But if the standard 50 mg of clomiphene citrate doesn't work, your doctor could jack up the dosage to 100 mg or 150 mg, which increases the cost slightly.

If clomiphene citrate doesn't do the trick, then infamous "injectables" are next on the checklist, and they get pricey fast. It comes as no surprise that this can range in cost between $2,000 and $5,000, depending on the specific drugs and dosages. These types of ovulation-induction protocols are often coupled with an IUI to increase the possibility that the sperm and egg meet.

Assisted Reproductive Therapy (ART) Medications

When ovulation induction alone doesn't work, things get a little more complicated. In general, medications used in IVF and other ARTs fall into three major categories. First, you will be prescribed some sort of gonadotropin-releasing (GnRH) analog. Either a *GnRH-agonist* or a *GnRH-antagonist* is used—each of which works in a slightly different manner to suppress the LH surge and ovulation until the follicles are mature. GnRH agonists typically are sold under the brand names Lupron, Zoladex, or Synarel—which is a nasal spray. GnRH-antagonists include Antagon and Cetrotide. Overall, costs for these medications range between $250 and $350 per cycle.

Next, gonadotropins are used. Typically, these contain some form of FSH (follicle-stimulating hormone), which is necessary to stimulate development of multiple follicles. These medications are extremely powerful and work directly on the ovaries to stimulate follicle growth. These medications include Bravelle, Fertinex, Follistim, and Gonal-f. Alternatively, medications containing both FSH and LH (luteinizing hormone) are used to stimulate the ovaries to produce multiple eggs in one cycle. Common FSH and LH combination medications include Humegon, Pergonal, Menopur, and Repronex. Given these are all highly potent medications that have to be injected over the course of several days or weeks, this is where you will spend the bulk of your medication dollars—somewhere along the lines of $2,000 to $5,000 per cycle.

Finally, hCG (human chorionic gonadotropin) is a single shot given at the end of your ovulation induction to cause final maturation of the eggs in the follicles. This will encourage the little egg to pop out of its nice comfy follicle to be either fertilized or retrieved. The common brand names for hCG are Pregnyl, Profasi, Ovidrel, and Novarel, and all cost about $50 or so. Additional medications that may be prescribed during an IVF cycle:

- Prenatal vitamins with folic acid
- Antibiotics for both male and female
- Oral contraceptives (birth control pills)
- Estrogen
- Baby aspirin
- Dexamethasone (a steroid that decreases inflammatory response)
- Insulin-sensitizing drugs (such as metformin) to help with problems like PCOS

Seems somewhat straightforward, right? Wrong! While all fertility medications fall into one of these major categories, there are many, many different ways they can be prescribed depending on your diagnosis and age, your doctor's experience and preferences, specific dosages, combinations of medications, and overall length of use. These types of variations contribute to whether you are on the lower or higher side of the price range. Let's look at how these decisions are made.

Deciding on a Protocol

Medication is a normal and necessary part of the IVF process, but it can still be complicated. If you don't get enough medication, your cycle can be canceled. If you get too much, you can develop ovarian hyperstimulation, and get canceled as well. As a rule, the fertility specialist reviews past stimulations, looks at the appearance of the follicles and your hormone levels to see how you are responding, and adapts accordingly.

"We tend to get a little superstitious about our IVF protocols," explains Dr. Sam Thatcher, director of the Center for Applied Reproductive Science (CARS). "Often, we use the same protocol we did when we were in medical school, as long as it is reasonably successful. Some doctors fear change. The other end of the spectrum is the doctor who jumps on the bandwagon and follows exactly what the hottest program is doing. Somewhere in the middle is the answer. I like for patients to be involved. The more they know, the more I appreciate it."

While some doctors may joke about consulting a Magic 8-Ball to decide about choosing a medication protocol, most doctors have their tried-and-true favorites. But that doesn't mean you can't be an informed participant when medication is being prescribed.

After all, this is your body. Your cycle. Your money. You have the right to not only understand your particular protocol, but also to be able to discuss why it's the best protocol for your particular situation. Regardless of what your physician may say, there is no perfect protocol.

Getting Involved

While your physician will factor in his or her experience with certain medications, and to some extent your particular circumstances, there is nothing wrong with bringing up the issue of finances as you are discussing your protocol. "Docs get in a habit of prescribing the same drugs all the time because they like the sales rep or that company funds their research," explains Toni Sarigosa, an infertility financial planner. "So don't be afraid to tell the doctor what your insurance covers and get them to go with your program. Maybe Ferring's medications are covered at a higher rate than Organon's, so you can save $200 out of pocket."

If your doctor has prescribed specific brand name medications, your pharmacist cannot change it to a lower-cost version of the same medication, although some unscrupulous pharmacies may try to do so in order to increase their market share of that particular drug. Any negotiations must be done with the doctor before you leave the office.

Once you begin reading magazines and websites dedicated to infertility, you'll be swamped with advertisements from the different drug manufacturers. Most of the ads feature a smiling baby, and all of them are intended to capture your attention and medication money. Since there isn't one perfect protocol, be aware of how you are being manipulated. Work with your doctor to make the best choice for you.

When you get your prescription, you can choose to have all of your prescription filled at once, but you risk having your cycle canceled and having a new protocol next month. Or you can wait until you need it to get it filled, but you'd better have a backup plan because mail order can be iffy and there is no guarantee anybody else will have it in stock. Patient-friendly pharmacists recommend that if a patient is paying out of pocket, to get only the first seven or so days of their protocol in case their therapy changes, and the

THE PHARMACEUTICAL INDUSTRY
WANTS YOUR MONEY

Pharmaceutical companies paid over $300 million to major PR companies to help them market their drugs.

- 95 percent of pharmaceutical advertisements used emotional appeals to sell medications, often framing them as a means to regain lost control over some aspect of life.

- 58 percent of pharmaceutical advertisements portrayed drugs as a medical breakthrough or as "new and improved."

- Some patient advocacy groups receive over 80 percent of their funds from drug makers.

From Melissa Healy, "Next Step: Create the Demand," the *Los Angeles Times*, August 6, 2007.

dose is either increased or decreased. This way, you are not left holding medication you don't need and can't return.

Extra Costs

A good deal of the medications you will be using will need to be injected. Since you aren't just downing a pill or two, this raises the complexity. Your fertility clinic is not going to do the injections for you, so don't even ask. They are too busy to even try to keep up with the injections of hundreds of patients. Most of us aren't in the habit of injecting ourselves several times a day. We all must learn how to do this correctly or find a willing helper.

A few doctors' offices capitalize on this and charge you to attend a "how to give yourself an injection" class. In our opinion, this should be included in the thousands of dollars you are already spending at their clinic. If they try to get you to pay this additional cost, speak up and they may be more likely to waive this one. If you are using a boutique pharmacy that specializes in fertility meds, it can be a good source of information as well. And don't be shy about enlisting the help of family and friends who are health care providers. There are even a couple of "How-to" videos posted on YouTube—one fertility patient trying to help another.

Your Insurance Company

"I was on Clomid and Menopur this month and I was shocked to see how expensive the Menopur was. When I asked my doctor for suggestions, he said I needed to go to a local specialty pharmacy about an hour from my house. They offer Menopur for half the cost, but my insurance doesn't cover the specialty pharmacy. No worries. All I had to do was check with the local grocery store pharmacy, which my insurance does cover, and they matched the prices of the specialty pharmacy."

—Lily

If you have insurance coverage for your medications, you still have to play an active role in getting the best deal. Your insurance plan may have a drug formulary, a list of prescriptions your health plan has approved. If a drug isn't on the formulary, you'll have to pay more for it. Your insurance company can give you a list of drugs on the formulary. Bring the list with you to the doctor's office. The list is usually effective for the calendar year, but it does change, so you want the most current list.

If you are fortunate enough to have drug coverage, get as much of the medications you need in one shot so you will make the most of a single co-payment. Otherwise, you could end of paying hundreds of dollars worth of copayments for one month of medications.

Your insurance formulary often depends on kickbacks your health plan receives from drug manufacturers. Manufacturers give incentives to pharmacy benefits managers to encourage certain medications be added to their formulary.

Where to Go

When most of us get a prescription, we just head on over to the nearest pharmacy or grocery store without a second thought. It really doesn't matter where we get our meds. Or does it? When it comes to infertility medications, you better believe it does. Most local pharmacies do not carry fertility medications, especially the injectables. Even if they do, they might not have the dosage you need or the expertise to provide you with accurate information on how to administer it. Finally, prices vary from pharmacy to pharmacy. Since we are talking about thousands of dollars here for medications, a little bit of a price difference can turn out to be a lot. Let's look at some of your options.

It Pays to Shop Around

EXAMPLES OF PRICING DIFFERENCES BETWEEN PHARMACIES

Pharmacy	Ovidrel PreFilled Syringe 250 mcg (a recombinant hCG-choriogonadotropin alfa injection or a recombinant hCG)	Gonal-f RFF Pen 900 IU (an FSH-follitropin alfa injection)	Cetrotide 3 mg (a gonadotropin-releasing hormone antagonist, cetrorelix acetate, for injection)
Freedom Drug	$44.25	$657	$359
IVFMeds.com	$60	$635	$440
FertilityMeds.com	$65	$779	$455

Prices checked 01/29/08

Your Clinic's Pharmacy

"I was so overwhelmed as I was leaving the fertility clinic, I was really tempted to just tell the fertility clinic to go ahead and give me the drugs while I was there. But I'd heard I should shop around first. I'm so glad I did! The cost at my Dallas clinic was $3,500; but I saved almost $500 going online."

—Layni

Some fertility clinics have a pharmacy as part of their practice, which is clearly convenient. It may not be cost effective. Somebody has to pay for the pharmacist, so it will get added to your bill somewhere. A portion of the medications you need may be cheaper there than anywhere else, but don't assume so. Do your homework first. One advantage of a clinic pharmacy is its return policy is usually fairly lenient and it will refund your money for unopened packages (although this is technically illegal). To encourage patients to utilize their internal resources, some clinics that offer a pharmacy on site will penalize you up to $250 for buying your drugs elsewhere. So ask about this before you buy your medications elsewhere.

LOCAL DRUGSTORES

Supporting local business is good, but sometimes it just isn't cost effective. We found it was difficult to even get infertility medications in a timely manner from local chain drugstores. Unless you live in an upscale market, they aren't going to carry vials of hCG, not to mention forty vials of gonadotropins. Don't assume they are going to have what you need when you need it.

In addition, chains can rarely negotiate prices and may be very ignorant about fertility treatment protocols. If excellent patient service and knowledge about the medications is important to you, don't shop there.

SPECIALTY PHARMACIES

There are a number of smaller, independent pharmacies that specialize in infertility medications. Often located in urban areas with more than one fertility center, they can be another source for fertility medications. William York, coowner of Concord Pharmacies, a chain of specialty fertility pharmacies in the Atlanta, Georgia, area, recommends that patients factor in service and knowledge of product when choosing a medication provider. "If you're only going to save two hundred dollars by choosing a local pharmacy over mail order, you need to carefully consider your options. When you're looking at a $12,000 IVF and $4,000 on meds, $200 is not a lot of money. The knowledge we have and the counseling we provide can and have saved a cycle and is worth more than that $200," says York.

There are some good reasons to spend a few extra dollars on a specialty pharmacy if you have one in your area. Knowledgeable pharmacists familiar with particular physicians' practices know what those practices run different protocols for and why this is important.

Explains York, "I had a patient several years ago who went to [a chain drugstore] to get her IVF meds—the kind that had to be done intramuscularly. She was assured by the pharmacist that they would have everything she needed. On the third day of the cycle, the pharmacist told her he couldn't get the promised meds and with those he did have, he gave the wrong instructions and wrong syringes. This was their one and only chance with IVF and she was petrified she had ruined her one chance.

"A very visibly distraught woman and her equally distraught husband came in, and I sat them down in our counseling area and calmly went through the bag of meds she had been given. I changed the errant syringes and needles they had been given as well as supplied her with the medications she would need for the rest of the cycle. The day after the successful retrieval, we got a huge arrangement of flowers. Twin boys came from that one cycle they almost lost. All because the pharmacist did not know what he was talking about and not only had no idea, but no initiative to call the doctor with medication questions."

In addition, York says, "Overnight delivery isn't guaranteed by the mail order companies. They try for it, but I get calls every single week from patients whose mail order medication is either wrong or not on time. If you get stretched to needing gonadotropins on the eleventh day and they can't get it to you in time, it's the worst kind of patient care. If you don't have it on hand, you might lose a cycle."

Smaller independent pharmacists do have the ability to negotiate, and you can always ask. "Sometimes patients will come in and ask if I can match a particular price. Occasionally I will," says York. "It depends on the situation and, sure, I'll do what I can, but I'm not going to go below cost. I don't want to make her pay for the sins of the drug industry."

POPULAR SPECIALTY PHARMACIES FOR INFERTILITY MEDS

Eveready Drug: www.evereadydrug.com
Freedom Drug: www.freedomfertility.com
MDR Pharmaceutical Care: www.mdrusa.com
Schrafts Pharmacy (part of Walgreens): www.walgreensspecialtyrx.com/infertility
Village Pharmacy: www.villagepharmacy.com

CHAIN DRUGSTORES

Prenatal vitamins, metformin, estradiol, progesterone, antibiotics, Clomid—all of these can be yours for only $4 at Wal-Mart. They are never going to add the injectables to their list of $4 medications, and you have to be able to pick them up in-store, but you can save several hundred dollars by getting the rest of your ART prescription filled at Wal-Mart or Sam's Club. In addition, they have special prices for clomiphene citrate and some birth control pills. You only save money if you don't walk out of the store with $50 in junk you don't need. When you go to your appointment, carry the newest updated Wal-Mart pharmacy list with you (available from any Wal-Mart pharmacy) to the doctor's office.

Online Pharmacies

For the last several years, the best way to save on infertility medication was to go to one of the online pharmacies specializing in infertility. For the big bad gonadotropins, this was particularly true. Sometimes, drug companies will limit your ability to make choices. For example, if you need Gonal-f, and you're paying out of pocket, Serono gives the deepest discounts only to one pharmacy. Therefore, you don't have many choices about where you'll get your meds unless you want to pay more—a lot more.

There are reputable legal online pharmacies, and they may be a way for you to save money. They work the same way a regular local pharmacy does, only the medications are shipped to your door. Some pharmacies offer free overnight delivery, while others don't. And those who offer free delivery may still make you pay shipping and handling for weekend deliveries.

There are the hidden costs, and you must read the fine print. Some mail order companies will charge a fee to join their service. It's bogus and pure profit. If you want to use their company, tell them you won't unless you drop that fee. The same thing goes for those extras like syringes and sharps containers. You can negotiate having those included in your package. If the customer service rep you are talking to can't do it, ask to speak to his or her supervisor.

Mail Order Programs

If you have medication coverage with your insurance, the insurance company may require you to use its mail order program. The big danger here is they can override your prescription and change it at will. Also, it may take three to four days to get approval. Again, by moving up the bureaucratic ladder, you may be able to negotiate being able to use a local pharmacy for at least the first month's cycle and/or get an immediate emergency approval.

Your fertility specialist may have certain "deals" with specific pharmacies or other agencies. Be sure to ask if there are any specific places you would need to purchase your medications. Asking other fertility patients about their drug-shopping ventures can also help you avoid pitfalls.

The following tips will help protect you if you buy medicines online.

KNOW YOUR SOURCE

A website needs to be affiliated with a state-licensed pharmacy located in the United States. Pharmacies and pharmacists in the United States are all licensed by a state's board of pharmacy. Your state board of pharmacy can tell you if this is a website for a state-licensed pharmacy that is in good standing and is located in the United States. Find a list of state boards of pharmacy on the National Association of Boards of Pharmacy (NABP) website at www.nabp.net.

A REPUTABLE AND SAFE PHARMACY WEBSITE SHOULD

- Be located in the United States;

- Have a licensed pharmacist to answer your questions;

- Require a prescription from your doctor;

- Provide access to a customer service representative person 24/7;

- Have a VIPPS Seal of Approval indicating they abide by strict standards and are a National Association of Boards of Pharmacy Verified Internet Pharmacy.

Why Are These Meds So Expensive?

Serono, Organon, and Ferring are the three big producers of infertility medicines. Ask any pharmaceutical rep at these companies why their drugs are so expensive and they'll follow the party line all the way to the bank—

research and development. Part of the reason drugs are so expensive is because their makers are trying to recoup their investment on years or decades of research and development that led to their creation.

The bottom line is these drug companies are in the business of making money. In the most recent year reported, Serono's sales rose by 31 percent to $519 million. That's how much medicine they sold. Its profits were $390 million. In other words, 75 percent of the cost of your medication is profit. To be fair, they aren't any worse than other players in the industry. But it doesn't mean it's compassionate care, either.

How to Save Money

There isn't much that can be done to offset some of these high costs for medications. If you are going through infertility treatments, the medications are a must. But there are things you can do to save a few dollars here and there. And we are big believers that every little bit helps.

Ask Your Doc for Freebies

"Some wonderful, fabulous, generous people donated their unused unopened fertility drugs back to their fertility clinic a few months ago. I was the very grateful recipient of donated meds. Our insurance doesn't cover any treatment for infertility and paying out of pocket is practically impossible for us. Paying for full cycles, we'd have been able to try once. By receiving donated drugs, we will now be able to try two to three times, which isn't a lot, but means everything since that first cycle failed."

—Tara

Doctors' offices sometimes have fertility medication waiting for a good home. Pharmaceutical reps give doctors free samples to be given away at the physician's discretion. Plus, if you're lucky, some doctors will accept leftover medications and redistribute them to other patients, as long as the drugs are unadulterated and are not controlled substances. All state boards of pharmacy as well as the FDA discourage it, and most lawyers recommend against it, but most brave doctors are willing to take the risk to help their patients.

Know Your Pharmacist

Pharmacists are the most underutilized health professionals. Where else can you get free information without an appointment? You will be taking a lot of medications during your treatments. Take advantage of all your pharmacist can offer. Don't hesitate to walk into your local pharmacy at any time and ask the pharmacist questions about your medications—how they work, possible side effects, how to administer them, if there are cheaper alternatives, and of course, why they may not be working. After all, it's your dime (or in the case of fertility meds, a whole lot of dimes)!

Investigate Pharmacy Programs

We know you're ready to get started pumping yourself full of hormones the second your feet are out of the stirrups. After all, who wouldn't want to inject purified urine from a postmenopausal woman into her tummy? (Actually, fewer drugs are made of urine now and are instead recombinant therapies.) But don't go running to the corner drugstore with your brand-new shiny script burning a hole in your purse. You need to understand the different types of pharmacies.

Once you know what drugs your insurance covers (ha!) and which ones your doctor wants you to have, then you need to learn who the manufacturers are, because all three infertility drug companies have deals with preferred pharmacies. In other words, they each have a guaranteed lowest price provider.

Serono works with Freedom Pharmacy (www.freedomdrug.com). Ferring works with a company called q.d.CARE (Commitment for Affordable Reproductive Endocrinology)—although, unbelievably, they don't have a website, your doctor might have the phone number. Organon works with DesignRx (www.designrx.com). While those dealers are supposed to offer the best prices, confirm by calling around.

Following is a list of FDA-approved fertility drugs and their manufacturers. If you are one of the lucky few whose insurance covers infertility medications, then they will generally cover only those that are FDA-approved for infertility treatment. It may also be helpful to know this information so you can track down which company offers which.

FDA-Approved Fertility Drugs

TRADE NAME	GENERIC NAME	MANUFACTURER	TELEPHONE NUMBER
Chorionic gonadotropin	Chorionic gonadotropin	Steris	602-278-1400
Chorionic gonadotropin	Chorionic gonadotropin	Fujisawa	847-317-8800
Novarel	Chorionic gonadotropin	Ferring Pharmaceuticals	888-337-7464
Pregnyl	Chorionic gonadotropin	Organon	800-631-1253
Clomid	clomiphene citrate	Hoechst Marion Roussel	816-966-5170
Serophene	clomiphene citrate	Serono	800-283-8088
Follistim	Follitropin beta	Organon	800-631-1253
Gonal-f	Follitropin alpha	Serono	800-283-8088
Ganirelix	Ganirelix acetate	Organon	800-631-1253
Repronex	Menotropins	Ferring	888-337-7464
Crinone	Progesterone gel	Serono	800-283-8088
Endometrin	Progesterone vaginal insert	Ferring	888-337-7464
Menopur	Human Menopausal Gonadotropin	Ferring	888-337-7464
Bravelle	Follicle stimulating hormone (FSH)	Ferring	888-337-7464

FIND DRUG COMPANY ASSISTANCE PROGRAMS

"My wife and I had recurrent miscarriages, and we could only afford one more fresh cycle. She wrote to the company who manufactured one of the medications, explaining why we could not afford it—and they sent her a six-month supply."

—DON

Most infertility drug companies have some form of financial assistance program available. These vary widely from company to company. Some are awarded on a first-come, first-served basis, while others are based strictly on need. Each program has a different set of guidelines, which may include who can be in the program based on several factors. These factors may include your income, age, diagnosis, number of previous cycles, and so on. These programs may change over time, so contact them for the latest information.

Serono has two such programs. If you are using Gonal-f, then Serono has basically strong-armed you to place your order through Freedom Pharmacy, unless you enjoy paying hundreds more for the same medication. The only redeeming factor is their Fertility Assist program. If you are paying cash and purchasing Gonal-f though Freedom Pharmacy, then Fertility Assist offers a discount on all Serono fertility medications to eligible patients for their second ovarian induction or IVF cycle. The second cycle has to be within eighteen months of the first and the amount you save depends on how much Gonal-f you use. If you are interested, ask your health care provider to enroll you.

In addition, Serono offers little-known medication scholarships called Compassionate Care, which gives away millions of dollars in free drugs to families who cannot afford fertility treatment. You have to go through an initial telephone benefits screening and you will need to provide a photocopy of your insurance card, two pay stubs, copies of your most recent tax returns, and be a US resident. If you are chosen, this program entitles you to one free lifetime cycle.

Ferring does its charitable duty by providing infertility patients with five free vials of Bravelle, a type of FSH medication, in its HEART (Helping Expand Access to Reproductive Therapy) program. When prescribing Bravelle, doctors need to attach a Bravelle HEART sticker on the prescription for you to take to a participating pharmacy. Infertility patients are pro-

---

CONTACT INFO FOR DRUG COMPANY
ASSISTANCE PROGRAMS

Serono 1-866-538-7879
Ferring Pharmaceuticals 1-888-337-7464 or email HEART@Ferring.com

vided with five free vials of Bravelle as part of a prescription of fifteen vials or more—a $300 savings. Or you can double your savings by purchasing thirty vials or more of Bravelle and get ten vials free—a $600 savings. Either way, you can also get a free box of Endometrin (a progesterone supplement), a $100 value.

Explore Other Discounts

"The Automobile Association of America (AAA) is great. I used them and got a prescription for Clomid 100 mg for five days and it would have been $50, but with the AAA discount it was $25. I also bought Provera/progesterone pills for seven days, it would have been $10, with AAA discount it was only $6. This is almost a 50 percent discount. With everything we're going through, any penny saved helps!"

—Becca

Check out what's in your wallet. You might be able to save money with memberships you already have. For example, AAA offers 5 percent to 20 percent discounts on your prescription drugs. When you are comparing prices, ask about those deals as well.

Shop Around

"The best advice I received about fertility meds was that you don't have to get all your meds from the same pharmacy. I called them and got price quotes. By using two different ones, I saved over $500, plus my fertility clinic had some donated meds from someone who had leftover. All I had to do was ask."

—Janey

Do your homework to find the best prices. The price tag can vary by $100 or more—per prescription. Whatever you do, don't get distracted by inconsequentials. Some pharmacies give the needles for free, but sometimes the pharmacy with the best prices charges for needles. Don't waste $50 to save $2.

Preferred-customer and discount programs at local pharmacies can make a difference as well. "The $12 VIP fee was an optional purchase giving you a discount on certain meds," explained Susan. "But by paying the $12 VIP membership fee, I saved about $500 on medication costs."

What About Leftovers?

*"A friend of mine asked the doctor to write the prescription for
the gonadotropins for the largest possible dosage—sixty ampules,
knowing she would need about half of it. Her insurance only made
her pay her copay and she could sell the other half of the meds to
defray the cost of the IVF the insurance company wouldn't pay for."*

—Tammy

You may be tempted to sell your leftover medications to someone else in the same boat. The problem is even giving drugs to other people is illegal. What if you don't respond well to a given medicine, but you change protocols for the next cycle? Is there a way to get your money back? Some fertility clinics with on-site pharmacies will allow returns of unopened boxes. Most places won't because of the threat of tampering and contamination, and the law is very clear—it can't be restocked for resale.

A Dirty Little Secret

*"I had one chance for IVF. We could only do it one time. We saved
enough to pay for the procedure, but there was no way we could
afford the $4,000 for the medications. The only way I could try it
was to buy the meds from someone else. But I was careful. I didn't
buy from the first person I contacted. It took a couple weeks, and I
ended up buying from the seventh person I talked to. I trusted my
instincts and kept on looking until I found someone I could talk to
on the phone for over an hour. By the time I finished talking to her,
I trusted her. I would do it again in a heartbeat."*

—Jayne

If you could buy fertility meds on the street corner and save 50 percent, most of us would. Do a quick internet search for popular fertility drugs, and you'll find a variety of purchase options within seconds. Thousands of women across the country trade or buy fertility drugs from other patients via the internet. Popular infertility bulletin boards, online auction sites, and even local support groups offer plenty of opportunity for such transactions.

What's the problem? Supply and demand, right? You've got a need and they've got leftover meds. But there are a few glitches. First, there's that pesky law thing. As pharmacist William York explains, "It's really clear: federal law prohibits transfer of drugs to any person other than for whom it was intended. That is the law. If it is a script-only medication, in order to be able to sell it, you need a license to sell it.

"Do they do it? Damn right, they do. But there are real risks—you don't know where the drug has been, where it has been stored. You don't know whether it is still effective or not. People will lie or cheat or steal all day long. I have not heard of anyone ever being prosecuted. There's hardly any way to police it with all the other stuff going on online."

Just because we don't know of anyone being prosecuted for buying or selling fertility meds online doesn't mean it can't or won't happen. In addition, a lawyer and a jury would have a field day deciding damages against the seller in the event personal injury or death was caused by the medications.

We hate to be the bearer of bad news, but purchasing fertility medications from online auctions or classified ads is like playing the lottery. Is it possible to find honest, straightforward people who are genuine and trustworthy? Absolutely. Could you also find someone willing to defraud you and cheat you without blinking an eye? Ditto. We know it's tempting to save money, but you don't know what you are getting, how it's been stored, or where it came from.

What if you get the wrong medication, medication that has expired or not been stored properly, or no medication at all? You have little recourse. You've got no one to turn to if you never get that precious package. After all, it's illegal to sell (or buy) the drugs in the first place. You could ruin your entire cycle if the medication is worthless and you don't know it. ART cycles don't grow on trees, and you're working too hard to get to yours, so don't throw yours away to save even a couple hundred bucks.

But what if you feel that the only option you have is to buy secondhand medications? If they are a legitimate source (someone from your doctor's office, a friend of a friend, and so on), then it may be a risk you are willing to take.

ORDERING INTERNATIONALLY

It is possible to order your infertility medications from another country and save money. It just isn't recommended. Those pesky FDA regulations make it tricky. Their position is this: virtually all shipments of prescription drugs imported from a pharmacy outside the country by a US consumer will violate the law.

Up to two million packages containing prescription drugs enter the United States through the mail every year, many of them as internet purchases, according to the FDA. Of those, fewer than 20,000 are detained and the addressees are notified that the products appear to violate the federal Food, Drug, and Cosmetic Act. If a drug is detained, the FDA is required by law to send you a written notice asking whether you can show that the product meets legal requirements. If you can't, the drug can be destroyed or returned to the sender.

Obviously, most packages aren't checked and you won't go to jail for trying to get your prescription filled in another country. But you might not get them, either. And just like buying leftover meds from another patient, you might not have much recourse if they don't deliver.

Lynn Blouin, a Canadian pharmacist who specializes in infertility medications, rarely has success filling US orders. "Sometimes very small packages will go through. If they are returned to me in a timely manner, I can give a refund, but not if they are damaged or expired. Sometimes the packages just disappear."

The FDA warns that those who buy drugs from foreign online sources risk getting fake, unapproved, outdated, or substandard products, with little or no quality control. Consumer advocates advise internet drug buyers to stick to sites in countries with the same pharmaceutical standards as the United States, such as Canada and European Union nations.

Pharmacist William York warns, "Several years ago, cases of counterfeit infertility drugs—with the same vial, same packaging—came from outside the United States. Patients thought they were getting a great deal, but there were no drugs in them. They looked perfect, and there was no way to tell they were fake.

"So, yes, you can buy them from London, Mexico, Italy. But you have no idea where they came from. Drugs in the United States are FDA-approved. If so, they are guaranteed to have what they are supposed to in them. If there is a bad batch or a drug recall, you have recourse through the courts or the manufacturer to make it right. If you don't know where a drug came from or and something goes wrong—you're screwed. People know it happens, but they don't think it will happen to them."

Pharmaceutical shipments discovered in "international mail" are referred to the FDA for examination. If you have ordered prescription drugs from an overseas source and have been told by either the courier service or the post office that they are being held, and you want to know about the status of the shipment, you can contact the FDA. We're not exactly sure what good it does to confirm your drugs are being held hostage by the federal government, but it's your dime.

FDA

Division of Import Operations & Policy
15800 Crabbs Branch Way, Suite 118
Rockville, MD 20855
301-443-6553

BRINGING IN MEDICATION FROM OTHER COUNTRIES

As a US citizen you should carry your prescription with you and check any regulations to minimize the chance it will be confiscated and you will lose it altogether. If a bag or package arouses suspicion, customs will set it aside and contact the nearest office of the FDA or the Drug Enforcement Agency for advice on whether to release or detain the drug product. Even though your bag may not be checked, it is against the law not to properly declare imported medications to customs. Failure to declare products could result in penalties. Possession of certain medications without a prescription from a licensed physician may violate federal, state, and local laws. Prescription drugs should be stored in their original containers, and you should have a copy of your doctor's prescription or letter of instruction. For more information about the US Customs Service, visit the agency's website, www .customs.ustreas.gov. In virtually all instances, individual citizens are prohibited from importing prescription drugs into the United States.

Many of the medications go by different names in different places. Here are some examples:

Foreign Names of Popular Fertility Medications

MEDICATION	US NAME	FOREIGN NAME
Human Menopausal Gonadotropin (hMG) contains FSH + LH	Pergonal Repronex Humegon	Pertisol Menogon Merional Lepori
Urofollitropin (FSH)	Metrodin	Fertinorm
Urofollitropin, highly purified (FSH)	Fertinex	Metrodin HP Fertinorm HP
Follitropin alpha and beta (Recombinant FSH)	Follistim Gonal-f	Puregon

Five Things You Can Do Right Now

1. Get your current drug formulary and a predetermination of drug benefits from your insurance company (use the sample letter in Appendix 4).
2. Visit your closest Wal-Mart/Sam's Club to get the newest $4 RX program list.
3. Ask your clinic about medications donated by clients or sales reps.
4. Call to get information about drug company programs.
5. Arm yourself with your drug list and get several quotes for each medication from both local and online specialty pharmacies.

CHAPTER 9

Don't Settle for No:
Be Your Own Advocate

"There were lots of things I should have talked to my clinic about. First, they never gave any written instructions. And my memory is the pits. Once you get to your individual protocol, that's issued verbally. I learned to be a fast note taker or else I wasn't going to know how to stick it to myself later. But once I got home, I was a mess trying to remember all that they told me. It wasn't until it was all said and done that the lightbulb went off in my head—I could have spoken up. If you don't ask, you will never get what you want or deserve."

—MICHELLE

WORKING WITH THE HEALTH CARE system as a partner in your health care is a crucial aspect of overcoming infertility. Since there are so many confusing terms, various treatment options, and intense changes occurring both physically and emotionally, you must remain active to ensure you're getting the quality care you deserve. You have it in your power to get just that!

It's just a matter of knowing what to expect and knowing how best to work hand-in-hand with your doctor, your insurance company, and the rest of the health care system. This way, you can rest assured your questions will be answered, your needs carefully discussed, your options clearly explained to you, and your concerns addressed.

Although it might not seem like it, you are the boss. You are the customer for whom the services are designed exclusively. It's up to you as a patient to be aware of your needs and what you are willing to accept. In the past, when you didn't like what a doctor said or did, you might politely thank him or her, then complain to your best friend as soon as you got home. While it's easier to complain to someone else, now is the time to shift gears and recognize misunderstandings, confusion, or even disagreements as opportunities on the way to getting the best care possible.

Working with Your Doctor

"It was several unsuccessful years into treatment when we decided to pursue the research we should have done upfront. I quickly learned that the price boasted by my doctor as being the best in the area was, in fact, accurate. We were saving about $1,500 on each IVF cycle by comparison to other clinics in the area. Unfortunately, the monetary cost was not the only price we were paying. According to the CDC, there were three other clinics within an hour's drive with significantly better stats that surpassed those of my current clinic."

—Jenna

When Cycles Don't Work

"There's always this hope that next time, the treatment will work. Next time, we'll change the meds just a little or I'll be less stressed out or something—anything that might make the next cycle the big one. I keep hearing about women who got pregnant doing a slightly different protocol and I think, maybe that would work . . . It's like a Ferris wheel I can't seem to step away from."

—Lori

We all get depressed when a cycle doesn't work. And we easily get sucked into the mentality of "Let's just give it one more try! I just know it will work the next time." This can go on month after month and even year after year with no results. How do you know when enough is enough is enough? Two years? Four? When you're bankrupt?

Getting pregnant is not an exact science, and we all know stories of babies conceived on the seventh IVF. But it's not the norm, nor is it fiscally responsible. It is helpful to at least have some expectations from the beginning. Think ahead and plan out how many cycles you can realistically handle physically, emotionally, and financially. You should never go in with the assumption that the sky's the limit. It is hard to know when to stop and it's even harder if you haven't fully thought it through beforehand.

To make the most out of your overall fertility plan, you must step back after each cycle, look at the situation objectively, and carefully consider your next step. It's kind of like sitting down after the game with the coach in the film room discussing each play carefully to find out exactly what went wrong. Yes, you can sit there and wish you were on a different team, had a different coach, or even had better weather. But this isn't what's going to help you win the next game.

IVF doesn't always work the first time. It is not your fault. Be practical and ask the hard questions. Why didn't this cycle work? Is there anything that can be done differently next time? How do we know it's time to move on and try something else? It's easy to let our emotions and our desire to have a baby take center stage. Get the support and information you need so you can rationally explore all of your options when a cycle fails.

WHAT DO YOU MEAN MY TEST RESULTS ARE INCONCLUSIVE?

"When my doctor came back and said that I needed an HSG, I immediately asked her how much this would cost. She said about $2,000. Since my husband and I are both teachers, this was a lot of money for us. Over the next few months we saved and saved. Cutting back on just about everything just so I could have this test. Once we got the results back, the doctor told us that one side looked fine, but she didn't know about the other ovary and tube since she couldn't get a good picture. I asked her what this meant. And she said that she recommended that I have the test again—costing us another $2,000. What? No discount! This was not my fault. I did everything I was supposed to do, and now we didn't even get the results we needed."

—LUCY

Sometimes you just don't get the information you need from medical tests for a variety of reasons, both within and outside your control. This is very frustrating when all you want is answers so you can get going on treating the problem that is preventing you from getting pregnant.

For starters, understand what the test is for and how you need to get ready for it. Sometimes the doctor will give you specific instructions about what you need to do in order to get the best results. Follow these instructions to the letter and do everything possible to prepare yourself (and your partner if necessary) for the tests.

If you get back inconclusive test results, ask about why this is the case. Was the test performed at the wrong time or under the wrong circumstances? Was there an error in how it was administered? Is the clinic doing anything to correct these types of mistakes? What can you do next time to prevent this from happening again?

Since all infertility tests cost money and have a very good chance of not being covered by your insurance plan, don't be shy to bring up the financial impact. How much is it going to cost you to repeat the test? If the reason for the inconclusive test result lies beyond your control, what is the clinic willing to do to rectify this situation?

Mistakes happen, but you should not be expected to absorb all of the cost. Clinics might not be used to being called out on issues like this, but you should always feel free to bring up your concerns. If you can get them to acknowledge any mistakes and give you a break, this will do a lot for your finances, not to mention your psyche.

When You and Your Doctor Disagree

"My first IUI cycle, I was never told I had to give blood at every ultrasound appointment. I think I had three ultrasounds before they finally clued in to the fact I wasn't giving blood for an E2 measurement. No one told me. The nurse said the doctor should have told me, and he said the nurse should have. They both indicated I should have known. After all, didn't I notice all of the other women getting blood work done after their exams? I can't help but wonder if not having all the blood work didn't help lose that cycle."

—Pamela

Infertility requires intense effort on the patient's part. Since treatment spans not just months, but commonly years, we are not easy "in and out" patients. We give ourselves shots, not the nurses. We change our lifestyle to improve

TEN STEPS TO EFFECTIVELY RESOLVE
YOUR DISAGREEMENT

1. Act quickly (although you might need a brief cool-down period if you are furious).
2. Stay calm and remain polite.
3. Articulate your problem systematically and concretely to the person you are having the disagreement with.
4. Ask questions and expect thorough responses.
5. Keep detailed notes.
6. Be honest about your emotions.
7. Discuss your ideas and concerns, even if you feel awkward about it.
8. Work through the disagreement.
9. Ask for a written summary of findings, diagnoses, and recommendations.
10. Agree on an action plan and be flexible (when appropriate).

our fertility, we do our own research, we rearrange damn near everything in our lives to accommodate this project. A lot of our care depends on what we do outside the doctor's office and our understanding of what we're supposed to be doing.

But we still need the clinic staff to do what they are supposed to do. It costs too much, it takes too much time, it involves too many tears for anyone to take this lightly. Sometimes even the most successful clinics mess up. Even the best nurse forgets to tell you something important. And on a few occasions, even the best doctors don't make the right call.

What do you do when you don't agree with the way you have been treated or you find yourself in a difficult position? Don't bottle up resentments, deny you are angry, take out your anger on other people, or just whine about it. You can control the outcome of this situation. Recognize that small mess-ups do occur, and know how to separate these from serious issues that compromise good care. Constant complaining about every little thing isn't going to get you very far.

Complain only to someone who can do something to address the situation. It is probably not effective to voice your frustrations to the receptionist or nurse. Always ask to speak to your doctor privately. Sometimes the setting can make a big difference. Confronting a doctor in front of staff is not the best tactic, nor is it appropriate to do so in the middle of the waiting room. Your doctor won't know you have a problem with your care unless you point it out. Doctors make mistakes too. And most doctors will want to resolve the problem.

If not, speak up. Ask to talk to the practice manager, write a letter, or file a formal complaint with your state's medical licensing board or the Better Business Bureau. In all aspects of health care now, the system and the doctors must be held accountable to the patient. It's your job to ensure this.

Second Opinions

In most cases where the medical condition and its treatment are complex, getting a second opinion makes perfect sense. But when you have to pay for all appointments, testing, and procedures yourself, it is difficult to know if a second opinion is truly necessary or financially beneficial. Becoming well educated about infertility issues will help you decide when a second opinion is needed. The best and most cost-effective time to consider second opinions is as early in your journey as possible.

Infertility is tough; we consistently get news we just don't want to hear. "Your follicles aren't growing." "Your hormone levels are out of whack." "This treatment is never going to work for you." This causes some of us to storm out of the doctor's office and seek someone else who might offer better news. More than one woman has gone to five or six or more clinics, desperate to find someone willing to take a chance on them. If you look hard enough, you will find someone who will tell you what you want to hear. But it may not be what you need to hear.

To save both your money and your sanity, look at the situation objectively and evaluate exactly why the doctor is saying what he or she is saying. If your doctor tells you that it just isn't financially or emotionally prudent to continue down the path you're on, listen carefully and ask lots of questions. What are the realistic chances for success and why? What other options are available that might have a better outcome? Is there a need to be more open-minded? As hard as it is, try to take emotions out of the equation. While it might not be your first choice, think long and hard about what is the best way to bring home a baby.

E-CONSULTS

With the advent of the internet, a few fertility clinics are taking full advantage of this technology by offering e-consults. For a few hundred dollars, you can send your medical records to another fertility specialist for his advice and insight. They will typically review your file and email you with a response. Occasionally, they will even agree to a telephone consult with one of their physicians. Prices range from about $150 to $300, depending on the extent and size of your medical record. And of course, you are also responsible for any related costs such as postage, copies, and telephone charges.

On his website, Dr. Mark Perloe, a fertility specialist practicing in Atlanta, explains that e-consults provide "reassurance that you seem to be on the right track, questions to ask your own physician, and access to the latest material about a particular medical concern." E-consults are not a replacement for in-person care, but if you are unsure about your diagnosis or treatment options, this might be simpler and more cost-effective than setting up a more formal second opinion (especially if you are going to need to travel to see another reproductive endocrinologist). This is still a relatively new idea, so you will have to do your homework and search out clinics that offer this service. If you find a clinic you like and they don't specifically state they do e-consults, bring it up as a possible option.

KNOW WHAT YOU'RE PAYING FOR

"After my IVF, I got an itemized list of charges from the clinic. I sat down with my bills and my calendar and I found three ultrasounds listed that I didn't have done. Catching that one error (times three!) saved me over $500. They sure weren't going to find it, and I can buy a lot of diapers with $500!"

—RENEE

Where else would you be expected to plop down $20,000 in cash with absolutely no information about exactly where this money will go? Fertility clinics should not be shy about providing a written itemized estimate of costs for your individual treatment plan. Still, most clinics will not provide this without you asking. Demand it even if they are reluctant to spill the beans. This will not only ensure you know how your money is being spent, but it will also preclude any unexpected charges. The itemized estimate should contain at least the following information:

- Pretreatment testing and evaluations (including both physical and mental health)
- Office visits, exams, and monitoring (how often, when, and why)
- Procedure costs (IUI, egg retrieval, embryo transfer, et cetera)
- Lab charges
- Doctor's fees
- Medication costs
- Information about how you will be notified of any treatment changes that will result in additional costs

There is always the possibility of emergency treatments that will add to

FERTILITY TREATMENT PLAN COSTS

In an online survey of 1,000 infertility patients, more than 85 percent paid privately. Of these, only 20 percent were provided with an individualized cost treatment plan, and the others were given general price lists or verbal information.

More than 25 percent experienced unexpected fees, and 88 percent would have preferred to have received a personalized fee breakdown.

the bill. But when you are paying for everything out of pocket, it's imperative you know the details about the expected and customary charges before you start. Documenting all this information will also put you in a much better position to negotiate with your insurance company about coverage of infertility-related expenses.

As soon as your treatment is completed, ask for an itemized account of all charges incurred. Using your calendar, confirm that all tests and procedures were actually performed in the manner explained and on the dates indicated. Billing errors do occur. Because you are paying for all (or at least a good portion) of the costs, it is up to you to find, note, and reconcile any discrepancies in a timely manner.

NEGOTIATE COSTS

We negotiate the prices of cars, our salaries, and even trinkets at flea markets, but negotiating with a doctor? Absolutely. Health care, especially infertility care, is a big business and there is wiggle room. According to a 2005 *Wall Street Journal* Online/Harris Interactive Health Care poll, only 12 percent of patients attempt negotiating with their doctor, but of those who do, 61 percent were successful in lowering their costs.

After all, health care providers negotiate fees and services every day with insurance companies, also known as "payers." These payers rarely pay the retail rate that the provider might want to charge, but instead negotiate with the provider until a mutual rate is agreed upon. So that exam you're being charged $150 for is costing the insurance company of the woman in the next room only $75 because that's the discounted fee your doctor has agreed to accept. While considered revolutionary in today's medical culture, it is reasonable to expect that no one is charged more or less for the same service.

You can negotiate with your clinic, but you must start the discussion. We guarantee that your clinic is not going to offer to negotiate with you. Lab work, anesthesia, and other fixed costs usually can't be talked down. But the costs of monitoring exams, ultrasounds, and administrative and instructional fees are all fair game. This is where your itemized estimate comes in handy.

Attorney and negotiating guru Michael Donaldson, author of *Fearless Negotiating*, urges couples to walk in the door of their clinic with a simple, straightforward plan to get what they want for the lowest price. He explains, "First, you must have as a core belief that you have other choices beyond the clinic you are in. You don't have to make a deal with just anyone. There are other places to go to." Make a list of the top three clinics you're willing to go to and get a list of their prices. Depending on geography, some have more options than others. Be open-minded and consider what you can do to save some money. Is a four-hour drive or a $200 plane ticket worth saving several thousand dollars? Your answer might be yes.

"Next, walk into your appointment, saying, 'I'll pay you 60 percent of what you're charging for IVF.' What the worst that's going to happen? He or she kicks you out? No. He might say he won't do it for that amount, but then you ask, 'Fine, then what can you do?' If he comes back with a 15 percent cut, then you counter with 25 percent and don't be afraid to say, 'We both know it's more than you get from an insurance company.'" Donaldson explains, "They have to have so many women in the pipeline to make money. Every now and then, they get a smart woman armed with a checkbook and a little bit of knowledge, and everybody wins. You get a lower price, and they don't lose money by accepting insurance negotiated rates.

"I took a national survey," jokes Donaldson, "and there were no fertility doctors who died of starvation. But many doctors are notoriously bad businesspeople. They are more likely to drop their fees in the fertility arena because they know they overcharge and there's plenty of competition. You have a lot of power if you can say, 'Thanks for your time, but Dr. So-and-so down the road will do it for $2,300 less.' It's not a threat; it's reminding the doctor you have alternatives." It is worth paying the initial consultation for two different doctors when you can potentially save thousands.

"You are not there to make a friend. You are there to make a baby. It's not a bad thing to negotiate. You're not powerless. You have a checkbook. That's power. You have choices. If 95 percent of patients always got a second quote for their infertility care, the prices would drop 40 percent across the country."

The most common mistake people make when negotiating is failure to establish a walk-away point. If the doctor makes an offer you think you might be able to live with, thank him or her politely and say you'll get back within a few days. Hit the pause button, go home, and let your emotions settle. If the physician pushes you to make a decision or establishes an arbitrary time frame in which the offer "expires," walk away.

The key to good negotiating is being prepared to establish your walk-away point. This may be more difficult for some than others. For instance, if you are older or have high FSH levels, it might be more difficult to find a clinic that will treat you, therefore limiting your options and your comfort level with walking away. We also know you want your doctor to like you. You want your doctor to be a source of support and encouragement, maybe even companionship along the way. But you don't have to roll over and be grateful to pay whatever a doctor asks. That 25 percent cut may make the difference in your ability to afford one more cycle.

TOP 10 TIPS FOR NEGOTIATING WITH YOUR DOCTOR

1. Talk to the doctor personally. Nobody else in their office has the power to negotiate.
2. Have the conversation face to face.
3. Bring a copy of the itemized estimate.
4. Ask for what you want clearly and directly.
5. Listen carefully.
6. Politely point out what other clinics have offered.
7. When hit with no, ask for what he is willing to do.
8. As difficult as it may be, put your emotions aside during this process.
9. When the doctor makes an offer, hit the pause button. Reply that you'll let him know in a few days.
10. Always thank your doctor for the time and consideration.

WHEN SOMEONE ELSE NEGOTIATES

There are a couple of companies out there that offer to negotiate with your health care provider for you. These companies call themselves health care discount programs.

Often, they focus on maternity benefits, but some are branching out to include fertility care as well. Typical plans cost a few hundred dollars up front and may also include a monthly fee or a percentage of the amount they end up saving you. In return, they offer to get you discounts by working directly with health care providers or buying services, such as lab tests or medications, in bulk in order to lessen the overall price. Unfortunately, you don't know beforehand how much, if anything, you will save. And there is no guarantee that your clinic or health care provider will be open to working with these types of programs. As a result, you might be forced to travel to another clinic, sometimes even out of state, to reap any benefits. While they may be able to get discounts for some people, there are far too many "if's" for us right now and no real guarantees of substantial savings. If you decide to go this route, ask lots of questions, including whether or not the discount program already has experience working with your particular clinic and with other patients who have had similar infertility diagnoses and proposed treatment plans. Don't be afraid to try to negotiate with your clinic yourself first. After all, you already have an established relationship with them so they might be more likely to work directly with you over someone else.

Working with Your Employer

Picture your insurance company as a used-car dealer. The dealer offers different types of cars to your employer, who, in turn, selects and provides a car to you. Your employer decides whether to offer you a cheap car with the bare necessities or the more expensive luxury car with all the bells and whistles. It is in the insurance company's best interest to offer the employer a wide variety of insurance options. If not, your employer will go to another "dealer." Your employer picks out your car—or policy, in this case,—including whether infertility treatments will be a covered service.

IT PAYS TO ASK

"I live in New York and my company didn't have to offer infertility benefits and they didn't. But I went to my employer and asked them to include an addendum to our current plan which allowed infertility coverage up to $10,000. That's for a lifetime, so it isn't great, but it's more than I had."

—EMMA

If your company doesn't have health insurance benefits that cover infertility, all is not lost. You still have options. First, ask your employer if the company would be willing to provide some type of coverage. Employers can choose to include an ART rider. More than five hundred companies have added infertility treatment to their health care plans just because someone asked! You haven't lost anything if you're told no, but they might surprise you. More and more companies want to become more family-friendly in order to attract and retain excellent employees.

Make an appointment to see your company benefits representative and come armed with information about the advantages and affordability of offering fertility benefits. Employers realize couples dealing with infertility are distracted by the physical and emotional hardships of this disease. The depression and emotional distress associated with infertility and its challenges have been clinically demonstrated to be equal to the psychological suffering of cancer patients. These high stress levels impact a person's general health, marriage, job performance, and social interactions—all of which ultimately impact the company's bottom line.

In 2006 Mercer Consulting, a highly regarded HR and benefits consulting firm, surveyed 900 US companies. It found:

- Over 90 percent said they had no increase in health care costs as a result of adding this infertility benefit.

- Over 20 percent of employers nationwide cover in vitro fertilization.

- Approximately 37 percent cover drug therapy for infertility treatment.

GET YOUR FAIR SHARE

Companies often offer different health insurance plans for different tiers of employees. In other words, the boss gets the SUV and the janitor gets the motorbike. For example, partners in the law firm may well have better, more thorough health insurance coverage than administrative assistants.

Liz Falker, a lawyer specializing in infertility, suggests making a discreet visit to your human resources office and asking if you could switch policies for a specific time period (a year, for example) and pay for the difference out of pocket. "One of my clients negotiated a better health care plan for two years. She had to pay an extra $200 a month and was sworn to secrecy, but it paid for all of her IVF treatment costs." Again, it doesn't hurt to ask.

Working with Your Insurance Company

WHEN PAYMENTS COME SLOWLY

Some insurance companies pay, they just take their sweet time about it. And if you're the one waiting to get reimbursed, or your doctor's office won't proceed until the insurance company pays, getting those claims paid on time may take some work. Go get your policy again and find out how long it says your company has to pay claims—generally it's thirty to forty-five days.

They must pay for your claim. We'll assume insurance companies want every bill paid in a timely and efficient manner, but they occasionally slip up. After every appointment, mark on your calendar the procedure and reimbursement amount, and then count ahead how many days the company has to pay out. Mark that date on your calendar as well. You already know what the insurance is supposed to pay because you have been so diligent beforehand, now it's just follow-up.

When the thirty days is up, check your records and see if you've received a claim form back. If not, call and politely inquire about the status of the claim. Check again the next day. And the next. Check until it's resolved the way your policy says it will be.

Don't assume the insurance company can add, either. If you have $1,000 deductible, then take responsibility for keeping a copy of every receipt, every bill, every penny you pay until your deductible is reached. That way, as soon as you've paid your portion and the insurance company should start picking up the cost, you'll be armed and ready in case their numbers don't match yours.

WHEN THE INSURANCE COMPANY WON'T PAY

"Insurance companies count on a margin of denials," says attorney Rhonda Orin. "They can't pay every claim. It is not in their interest to do so. From personal experience, if you do things a certain way, you are more likely to get a reversal of denials. Some couples write this impassioned, emotional letter, enclosing pictures of their houses and dogs and write about their loneliness. None of this matters to the insurance company. It is a business. This isn't personal to them. Even if you beg them, they can't cover you. You must approach them systematically. They do make mistakes. You can force them to deal with you."

How many times have you argued with your insurance company? Most of us don't because we assume they're right. The odds are, you have been unfairly turned down for a claim somewhere along the line. We all have. Exact numbers vary, but about 10 percent of all insurance claims are unjustly denied. How can insurance companies get away with it? It saves them money, because fewer than 1 percent of people making insurance claims even question their insurer when their claim is denied. According to Orin, the majority of policyholders who do contest their cases either win their cases or improve their settlements. How? Here are some tips to get started:

TOP TIPS FOR COPING WITH YOUR INSURANCE COMPANY

1. Develop a point of contact for all insurance issues and needs. A specific contact person within the insurance company will give you more responsiveness when discussing your claim.
2. Put everything in writing. Even if you call, follow up with a letter.
3. Include the claim number in every call and letter. Insurance companies process, file, and retrieve information by claim numbers, not individual names.
4. Understand the business of insurance. Your insurance company does not hate you, but it must limit claims to stay afloat, so your claim must be well supported.
5. Never threaten to cancel an account or take legal action unless you are willing to follow through. Insurers keep logs of all your telephone calls and letters. If you threaten the company with legal action, the claim may be turned over to their lawyers and may be delayed for much longer.

- **Insist on a written explanation.** Most state laws require insurance companies to provide written explanations of claim denials. Failure to comply may constitute an illegal practice by the insurer.
- **Do not accept filing errors as grounds for refusal.** Always follow your insurer's instructions for filing a claim. But if you fail to fill out a form correctly or if you miss a deadline for submitting a claim—even if you are months late—an insurance company cannot refuse to pay an otherwise valid claim unless the company can show it has been harmed by your error or prevented from making an adequate investigation due to your delay.
- **Ask your insurance agent or group policy administrator at work for support.** Your human resources department at work may be able to help you when a claim has been denied. If you purchase a policy individually, call the insurance agent from whom you purchased it. He or she has an ethical and legal responsibility to assist you so the coverage protects your interests.

"I was fighting with my insurance company about the claim, and bills were being sent to collection agencies for nonpayment. It was only after I requested advice from my benefits administrator at work on how best to handle this, that I found any help."
—Sandi

- **Keep great records.** Begin with the person who denied your claim, then write to the person's supervisor. Include your policy number, copies of all relevant forms, bills, and supporting documents and a clear, concise description of the problem. Request that the insurer respond in writing within three weeks. Keep copies of all correspondence. It creates a paper trail you'll need if it ever gets real ugly. If you receive no response, send follow-up letters, with your original letter attached, to the insurance company's consumer complaints department and to the company president. In most states, failure to respond promptly to letters regarding claims is an unfair insurance practice.
- **Request an appeal.** To file an appeal, you must find out what the internal process at your health plan is. Many states require that the

health plan have two levels of appeal. First, an executive appeals committee, usually consisting of a medical director, an employee, and a nonemployee, would review your claim. Basically they review the request and why the request was denied, always going back to what is covered in your policy. The decision is usually given to the member via mail within seven days. Some states have an additional external review process in which a committee outside the health plan will review the appeal. Find out at your state insurance website what they offer.

It's pretty clear-cut. If something is not covered under your plan, there's no getting around it. If you were told you were otherwise covered, bring as much info as you can. Who told you and when? How were you told? You need documentation for everything. If the procedure was covered a few months ago, but a change to your policy was made and it is no longer covered, you may be "grandfathered" in. You still may be able to get it covered if you can show that you were not properly notified of the change and already had the procedure scheduled. A health plan appeal information organizer is located in appendix 5 so you can keep all the information you need together.

- **Get your doctor in the game.** While your doctor's office may not do handstands at the opportunity to write a letter to your insurance company, they can (and should) do it for you. They must use the language of your policy in their letter. For example, if your policy allows for infertility coverage only in cases of "failure of Clomid challenge" or "elevated FSH numbers," then those terms must appear in your letter. Make a copy of the appropriate page of your benefit book and give it to the office with the right terminology highlighted. Offer to pick up the letter and mail it (certified, of course) yourself after you've made a copy for your records.
- **Read the decision letter carefully.** One woman's claim denial was based on the findings of the insurance company's own staff physician, who happened to be a board-certified neurosurgeon. His argument for turning her down for egg donation, which was covered by her policy, was that she failed the ovarian reserve test.

What? Of course she did, argued her attorney, hence the need for donor eggs. There are two lessons to be learned here: First, you have the right to have your case evaluated by a board-certified physician who specializes in reproductive endocrinology or gynecology. Second, question the answer because sometimes the denial will quote your policy wrong. Do not assume it's right.

• **Call for backup.** If you truly believe that the procedure, medication, or office visit should be covered because your policy says so, and your claim is denied, you may wish to contact your state department of insurance. While their help is free, the amount of help these departments can give varies from state to state. But some states with strong departments (such as California, New York, and Illinois) will mediate your dispute. A professional arbitrator or a lawyer is another choice, but they can get pricey.

Your Mother Was Right

Whether your fight is with your doctor's office, your employer's HR department, or your insurance company, there is one thing you must keep in mind: don't be a bitch. You might feel that you have a right to be, and you are probably spot-on with these sentiments. The situation sucks; people screw up; institutions make bad rules that don't make any sense and aren't fair; clinics sometimes care more about money than they do about people. It's enough to make a girl bitter. Don't go there. At least not when you're talking to the people who can help you.

You do get more flies with honey than with vinegar. So dial down the crazy and play nice (as much as humanly possible, that is). See each person as someone who wants to do the right thing and wants to be liked. Part of empowering ourselves to take charge is to enlist people who can help us along the way.

> *"I was fighting with my insurance company over a claim that I thought should have been paid. I decided it couldn't hurt to be nice to the insurance representative I spoke with, even though it was a stretch for me because I was annoyed and a little panicked about the $12,000 at stake.*

"I learned her name, thanked her for her help, asked what I could do to help her with the claim, and generally made sure I was the nicest customer she talked to all day. It took days and days of phone calls, but I always made sure I spoke with the same woman, and she ended up going to bat for me, and the claim was covered. If I had alienated her at the beginning, I'm pretty sure the claim would have been denied."

—Lindsay

Maybe Your Mother Wasn't *Always* Right

"I had major arguments with my insurance company during my infertility treatments. And I mean major! Still, I remained very combative. When the representative offered an arbitrary and unfair settlement, I told her I had to get off the phone now to call the investigative reporter at our local news channel about this consumer abuse. In about three minutes, I was given full payment. I can't say this was easy, but I am an attorney professionally trained in litigation. I know not everyone can do this, but if you can find it in yourself to pull it off, it's worth it."

—Mary Ellen

It's tough to know when to hang in and fight with all your might and when to give in a little. Some of us are better at this than others. If you like confrontation and you deal well with difficult situations, go for it. If it's not your strong suit, perhaps your partner is ready, willing, and able to do so and might welcome an opportunity to play a more active role in the process to take some of the pressure off you.

Keep in mind there may be consequences when you play hardball. Your doctor's office may decide not to keep you as a patient, or you might lose the battle with the insurance company. But the stakes are high enough that it may well be worth the risk.

When Not to Fight

Some battles aren't worth fighting. For instance, filing a grievance about medications rarely ends well. The medication benefits in your policy are usually clearly spelled out. They either pay for fertility medications or they don't. Although, if not, they may pay for some medications not exclusively used for fertility, such as birth control pills at the beginning of a cycle, or an insulin resistance medication if you have PCOS. Other than that, don't waste your time or energy with this type of complaint.

Likewise, there is no law stating your infertility doctor must treat you no matter what. Since infertility is not life-threatening, it's up to your clinic's discretion as to whether or not to keep you as a patient. You definitely have the right to speak your mind if you don't agree with or aren't satisfied with your care. However, if you become too belligerent, they aren't going to deal with you. While we don't agree with these types of situations, please know that some patients have been fired by their doctors simply for being too difficult to work with. Based on your own individual circumstances, only you can decide exactly how far you want to take your battle.

When Less Is More

After struggling with infertility for years, you might think you'd be thrilled to get two, three or even four babies for the price of one. It's tempting to transfer back as many embryos as possible. After all, if you transfer back ten, the chances of success increase tenfold, right? Not exactly.

The exact number of embryos that should be transferred during any single IVF cycle is open to debate but should never exceed four, and that's only for women with extenuating circumstances, such as multiple failed IVFs. Research shows transferring no more than four embryos per IVF cycle will yield optimal results.

Exactly how many embryos to transfer depends on a number of factors, including mother's age, stage of embryo development, and quality of embryo. Some reputable clinics are abiding by a "two-embryo transfer policy." As skills in the embryology lab improve and we learn more about what contributes to a successful implantation, professionals are beginning to encourage more single-embryo transfers.

Take this decision about how many embryos to transfer seriously and do not let anyone talk you into transferring more embryos than you should. Your goal is a single healthy baby. With a great fertility specialist and embryologist, transferring back just one or two well-developed embryos offers the greatest likelihood of at least one of them becoming a healthy baby.

If you transfer back three, four, or more embryos, you must be prepared to be pregnant with twins, triplets, or quads, no matter how small you think your odds. In fact, according to the CDC, 30 percent of ART pregnancies end up in a multiple birth. More than one practice has transferred two great-looking eggs that later divided and Mom had triplets. Likewise, if you go through with an IUI knowing you have several follicles and potential eggs available, prepare yourself for multiples. How many sextuplet stories have you seen on the Discovery Channel? You don't want to star in one.

Multiple-birth pregnancies are complicated. They necessitate more doctor's appointments, testing, bed rest, hospitalizations, and ultimately time away from work and other activities. This can result in lost wages and more money being spent on basic household assistance. Being pregnant with multiples can be dangerous to both mother and babies. The more babies you carry, the greater the chance you won't bring any home. You may also be faced with even tougher decisions like selective reduction, a procedure by which the number of fetuses is reduced.

Once the babies are born, expenses continue to escalate exponentially. Babies from multiple pregnancies are much more likely to be born prematurely and require neonatal intensive care. At least 50 percent of twins and nearly all other multiples are born prematurely, and the more babies you're carrying, the less time they have to "cook" in the womb. Babies born from multiple pregnancies represent 20 percent of all very-low-birth-weight infants and can develop serious and life-threatening complications. Premature births also result in higher rates of learning and developmental disabilities, including autism.

While insurance will start to pick up babies' expenses after birth, you will still be responsible for deductibles, insurance premiums, uncovered expenses, and more lost work time. And don't forget the extra help. With more than one baby born at the same time, you are going to need extra hands for all those feedings, diaper changes, cleaning, and waking up at all hours of the night. Unless you have a large supportive family living nearby, you are going to have to pay someone to pitch in.

During the first year of life, the medical costs of a single premature baby are more than $41,000 compared to about $3,000 for a full-term baby. If you have several babies requiring specialized care for long periods of time, this can easily top the $1 million mark. According to the March of Dimes, these high costs result in about $26.2 billion annually. And this doesn't even include lifetime health care costs for any premature-birth-related problems.

This makes the cost of an IVF cycle look like chump change. If the cost of infertility treatments were more reasonable, patients would feel less pressure to "push the envelope" to maximize their limited chances at having a baby. More money spent on the front end will ultimately save billions in the long run, resulting in healthier and happier families and employers alike.

Why Infertility Coverage Should Be Offered

"In one year, my insurance company spent about $25,000 on surgery, drugs, doctor's fees, and tests to diagnose and treat my endometriosis. If they have to, they'll jolly well do that every year until I hit menopause, making the bill for my treatment a cool half a million dollars. They won't, however, spend $11,000 on IVF, which, unlike trying "naturally," has a good chance of slowing the progress of the endometriosis, therefore actually saving my insurance company money in the long run. Let's see: $500,000 or $11,000. Tough choice."

—Susanna

It doesn't make sense. There are times when paying for ART would save insurance companies money. As we just mentioned, births of four or more babies are almost always the result of families trying less expensive types of fertility treatment—stimulation of egg production through drug therapy followed by an IUI—in hopes of maximum return. If the cost of IVF and other ARTs are so far out of reach, couples will go with the less expensive, yet sometimes more risky, procedures just to have a baby. As a result, some moms will have multiple low-birth-weight babies, whose short- and long-term medical care can easily add up to millions of dollars.

Here are also several other good reasons why infertility treatment should be covered by insurance.

INFERTILITY IS A TREATABLE MEDICAL CONDITION

Infertility is a medical condition. Almost 90 percent of the time, one or more specific medical causes can be identified. Some causes are structural abnormalities in the reproductive tract. Other causes are the result of a disease, such as cancer or endometriosis, or an endocrine disorder, such as PCOS. As such, infertility has much in common with other medical conditions that are caused by structural abnormalities, disease, or hormonal imbalances.

The Americans with Disabilities Act and the U.S. Supreme Court have confirmed that the ability to reproduce is a "major life activity," akin to seeing, walking, working, and caring for oneself. Within that context, a disability is defined as a physical condition that prevents someone from participating in a major life activity. For the majority of infertile couples, infertility is a treatable medical condition, for which nonexperimental, minimally invasive procedures, such as IVF and artificial insemination, are extremely effective if performed appropriately.

INFERTILITY TREATMENT IS MEDICALLY NECESSARY

Infertility treatment is absolutely medically necessary. Medically necessary treatment generally has to be: (1) safe and effective; (2) not experimental; and (3) appropriate. Treatment of infertility with IVF clearly meets these criteria, as IVF is safer, more effective, and less costly to the health care system compared to many surgical procedures, such as those for tubal reconstruction or removing endometriosis. These more expensive, less effective infertility-related surgeries are covered by most medical insurance while IVF is not. IVF is not experimental, it has been used for more than thirty years and is recognized by the American College of Obstetricians and Gynecologists and the American Society for Reproductive Medicine. Because it is less invasive, less risky, and more successful than alternate surgical approaches, it is often the most appropriate and sometimes the only appropriate treatment for infertility.

Treatment Will Lower Costs

Some health care providers oppose a federal mandate for insurance coverage of infertility because profit margins within the medical field may be reduced. For example, in Massachusetts, where coverage is guaranteed to all policyholders, insurance companies set limits on treatment costs. The consequence? Reduced profits to clinics and physicians. This all translates to more patients for less money if insurance is involved. And it's no secret—uninformed clients who pay doctors directly will almost always pay more. As a result, doctors are split as to whether they should support insurance coverage for infertility or not.

Take Dr. Mark Perloe. He explains, "Mandated coverage would simply mean that we would do a greater volume of IVF procedures, but we would have to limit the relationships we have with patients because we have to pay the bills. IVF is expensive, and most insurance companies barely pay enough to cover the cost of the procedure, and that's with no profit."

And yet there are other physicians who are vocal proponents for coverage. Dr. Sam Thatcher says mandated coverage is the right thing to do. "If physicians really care about patients, then he or she also really cares about financial well-being of patients as a stressor. Stress affects fertility. We know that. Every day I work with patients who make decisions about their care based on what they can afford. It needs to change."

Advocate for Insurance Reform

Belle Degenaars, the mother of two children—six years and several miscarriages apart—devoted four years to obtaining passage of the New Jersey Family Building Act. The law requires health insurers to provide coverage for medically necessary expenses incurred in the diagnosis and treatment of infertility. Her tireless efforts are responsible for thousands of families now having access to infertility treatment. States get mandated coverage only when passionate people get involved and start working with legislators to make it happen.

Few people would dispute that health insurance needs reform. Less than a quarter of all health plan sponsors with at least ten employees provide some level of coverage for infertility treatment. The cost of including a well-managed infertility benefit is minimal. Massachusetts, the state with the most comprehensive mandate for infertility coverage, found that the cost of coverage was one of the lowest among its mandated benefits, at $2.49 per member per year.

Nice girls don't fight, right? Sometimes they do. We need to fight for ourselves, for our checkbook, for our right to be heard, respected, and treated fairly. You have a lot at stake—the next cycle could be the one.

And even if it doesn't work out for you right now, we need to fight for the men and women who follow us. If you are willing to go to bat at work for infertility coverage or advocate at the statehouse, then families will have you to thank for years to come. "I wish I could explain how good it feels to meet parents who show me their children's pictures and tell me that because of me, they have a family," says Degenaars. You already know how hard this is. If you can find ways to make it easier for somebody else, then let your infertility journey bless somebody else. Besides, a little good karma can't hurt.

Five Things You Can Do Right Now

1. Organize your health insurance claim and policy information.
2. Start a calendar just for health insurance claims.
3. If your insurance is lacking, make an appointment to talk to your HR department about other options.
4. Check with our website (www.myfertilityplan.com) or the website of the other infertility patient organizations.
5. Actively support a bill requiring insurers to cover infertility. You'll find a sample letter to your legislator in appendix 7.

CHAPTER 10

I'll Try Anything!:
Investigate Creative Alternatives

"By the time we had been beaten by our fourth IVF cycle, we had already begged and borrowed from relatives, written checks from a home equity loan, and taken part-time jobs to supplement our income. We had squeezed every cent from our bank accounts and rummaged the couch cushions for spare change. Sadly, no one had dropped a check for $10,000 in the recliner."

—JENNA

WHOEVER SAID NECESSITY IS THE mother of invention must have been trying to get pregnant. The baby quest requires couples to think creatively and look for innovative ways to meet financial challenges. Wishful couples have a number of different options, from participating in clinical trials, changing jobs to a more family-friendly company, or moving to one of the few states requiring some employers to provide coverage.

Participate in Clinical Trials

Clinical study and clinical trial are the same thing—a scientific study of how a new medicine or treatment works on people, as opposed to in test tubes or in animals. Before these treatments can be prescribed, they must also prove safe and effective in humans. This kind of clinical testing is done on a volunteer basis only, and participants must understand the risks and benefits of taking part in a study. Most important, volunteers can leave a study at any time if they change their minds. Each clinical study tries to answer specific scientific questions and help doctors find new and better ways to prevent, detect, diagnose, control, and treat illnesses such as infertility.

You don't have to live near a university teaching hospital to take part. In one metropolitan area, a local fertility clinic was recently recruiting for three research studies. One study focused on determining whether it is best for a woman under forty years of age to limit the number of IUI cycles before moving on to IVF, another was trying to determine the best treatment for women between the ages of thirty-eight and forty-two, and a mind-body study investigated the impact that stress has on IVF outcome.

Participants in the studies won't necessarily get a full free ride, but a portion of treatment costs—sometimes a substantial portion—will be paid for. Often the medications and one IVF cycle are covered. But there are always risks, and you've got to do your homework. Brush up on your clinical trial knowledge and check for new trials often, because they fill up fast.

Before the FDA can consider an investigational drug or treatment for approval, it must be shown to be safe and effective in a clinical trial. Researchers follow strict ethical and scientific principles so patients are protected and valid results are produced. A plan of how the study will be run, or the protocol, is written by the study's sponsor. All researchers taking part in the study will use the same protocol. It describes in great detail how the study will be conducted: the number of participants to be enrolled, the amount of drug to be used, the types of medical tests to be provided, and other details of treatment.

To ensure patient safety, the protocol must be reviewed and approved by the organization that sponsors the study as well as by an institutional review board. This board consists of people with a variety of backgrounds and may include clergy, health professionals, and members of the general public. In the review of the protocol, the board seeks to ensure that participants in the study will not be exposed to unreasonable or unethical risks.

Compared to the number for cancer or heart disease, there are far fewer clinical trials for infertility, but physicians, pharmaceutical companies, and hospitals fund more than one hundred infertility-related clinical trials a year, providing several thousand men and women with free or reduced-cost treatment.

There are some drawbacks you need to consider. Experimental trials are just that: experimental. You have to take the leap of faith that the drug will work and that the side effects will be tolerable. In some cases you must also be prepared to be the one who is in the comparison group and does not get the intervention. It's a risk you need to know you're taking. You may still benefit from getting a more accurate diagnosis.

CONSIDERING A CLINICAL TRIAL?

The National Institutes of Health recommend asking these questions before participating in a clinical trial:

- What is the purpose of the trial?

- What kinds of tests and treatments are involved?

- What is likely to happen in my case with, or without, this new research treatment?

- What are alternative treatment options and their advantages and disadvantages?

- How might this trial affect my daily life?

- What side effects might I expect from the treatment?

- How long will the trial last?

- Will hospitalization be required?

- Who will pay for the treatment?

- If I were harmed as a result of the trial, what treatment would I be entitled to?

- What type of long-term follow-up care is part of this study?

Some clinical trials involve testing new treatment options. One example is egg freezing. Clinics are studying how to best achieve pregnancy with frozen eggs. While many clinical trials run by fertility clinics cost less than established treatments, the rates for success are generally low. Even if you get a 50 percent discount on the treatment, you're still paying for meds and your chances of success are not good. It is not fair to pay to participate in a clinical trial. The low odds are not worth the investment of your money. Save that money and put it toward a more established treatment or convince the clinic that participation in a clinical trial should be offered at no cost to the patient.

There are different kinds of trials for different phases of drug or treatment development. They are divided into types, called phases.

Phase I Trials

The first human tests of investigational drugs or therapies occur in Phase I trials. Phase I trials are designed to determine the best dose of the study drug and to check for any potential side effects. These trials usually involve small numbers of volunteers. Because Phase I trials use study treatments that have never been tested in humans, they can involve significant risks, but don't always. For example, the National Center for Complementary and Alternative Medicine (NCCAM), hypothesizing that acupuncture can significantly increase the IVF pregnancy rate, funded a Phase I study to examine the effect of acupuncture on IVF pregnancy rate.

Phase II Trials

If an investigational treatment is initially shown to be safe and well tolerated, it moves on to Phase II trials. These trials are designed to see how well the study treatment works, usually in a larger group of patients. An example of a recent Phase II study compared the effects of omega-3 fats plus folic acid with those of placebo plus folic acid on sperm quality and sexual function in infertile men.

Phase III Trials

If the investigational treatment is effective in Phase II trials, it may move on to Phase III trials. Phase III trials test how well the drug works in hundreds or thousands of patients. Phase III trials compare the study drug to an existing standard treatment, called the reference drug, in a randomized fashion. An example was a trial that attempted to determine the role of the medication DHEA on follicular dynamics in the human ovary and to better understand the interaction of DHEA supplementation with other treatments for ovulation induction among older women of reproductive age.

Phase IV Trials

These trials are conducted after a drug has been approved by the FDA and after the drug is on the market. Phase IV trials typically involve a large number of participants. They may evaluate new uses of existing therapies or be used to detect side effects not appearing during Phase III studies. For example, a recent Phase IV study examined the outcomes of various medication protocols during IVF in women who were expected to have a decreased response to ovarian stimulation. Another Phase IV study focused on women with polycystic ovary syndrome (PCOS) who ovulated with insulin-sensitizing medication but did not become pregnant. The study looked at the efficacy of controlled ovarian stimulation (COS) followed by intrauterine insemination (IUI).

SIGN ME UP!

ClinicalTrials.gov (www.clinicaltrials.gov) provides updated information about federally and privately supported clinical research on human volunteers. The website has information about a trial's purpose, who is eligible to participate, locations, and phone numbers for more details. Check with your clinic, too, to see if your physician is aware of any upcoming trials.

Clinical Trials: Medications

The major pharmaceutical companies that manufacture medication for infertility treatment conduct clinical trials for new products. Trial participants can receive free medication as well as free procedures. One study, for example, compared fertility medications in their ability to prevent spontaneous ovulation with ART treatment, and therefore significantly decrease the number of injections the patient receives with treatment. For information and to apply for other studies, visit the websites of the major infertility pharmaceuticals: www.ferring.com, www.serono.com, or www.organonusa.com.

Apply for an IVF Grant

"This grant made our dreams come true," says Yadira Campis and her husband Jaime Medina, fertility treatment grant winners and the parents of twins born from their free cycle. There are a handful of places that give out money for infertility treatment. Not many places and not to a lot of couples, but it does work for some people if they apply. And applying is work—all grant programs require a pretty extensive packet.

Not all IVF grants are created equal. Some are legit, while others are

COMMON INFERTILITY GRANT
APPLICATION REQUIREMENTS

- A 2- to 3-page application with basic personal information;

- A short essay describing your personal situation;

- Medical documentation supporting your infertility history;

- Tax records, pay stubs, and proof of financial need;

- Family photos;

- Letters of reference.

complete scams. How can you keep yourself from being ripped off? Some organizations require you to pay a membership or application fee of $50 to $100 just to apply. Having to pay some sort of fee because you need money rubs us the wrong way. Enough of the grants actually end up being scams, so guard your checkbook—and your private financial information. Seriously consider whether it is a reasonable investment to pay for a small chance for a grant.

Always check out the organization thoroughly before you send anything. Call directly and ask specific questions about the grant opportunity and application process. Questions should include: What are the application requirements? How is a decision made? How soon will we find out if we are chosen? How does the organization get the money for the grants? How will you be contacted about the results? What will the grant include? How many grants have been given out so far? If selected, what will be our responsibilities? If the grantor refuses to talk to you, be suspicious. Also, contact the Better Business Bureau in the state where it is located to find out its history.

Frankly, it's a long shot, and you may have better luck buying $50 in lottery tickets. But if you've got $50 in Christmas money from Grandma burning a hole in your pocket, go for it. Read the fine print carefully. For one grant, you still have to pay to travel to the participating clinic, buy your medications, and fund-raise for the organization. You may also be asked to sign away rights you don't really want to give up. For example, they may want to capture all aspects of your treatment on video and film to use your story for promotional purposes. Again, we think these are unfair prices to pay in exchange for a grant.

Likewise, fill out the paperwork very carefully. One organization requires a fee to resubmit if your application is incomplete. Not surprisingly, many of the applicants we talked to had to pay the resubmit fee. And most of these grant organizations don't accept phone calls or inquiries about the status of your application, so you better be extremely patient. It can easily take up to a year from the time you apply to the time you get the money, delaying your treatment even longer. Even under the best circumstances, you are still going to get stuck with some costs. Most grants will only pay for up to $10,000 to $15,000 if you are lucky. A grant can help, but don't expect a totally free ride.

Most important, when applying for a grant ask about the selection criteria. Keep in mind they are going to pick people who have a reasonable chance of success. In other words, if you are forty-five and using your own eggs or if you have had four failed cycles, don't expect a check in the mail. Likewise, these organizations are going to want promotional material appealing to the widest possible audience. Married, heterosexual couples stand a greater chance of winning than do single women and couples in different circumstances.

Although we like the concept of helping people out with financing treatment, all of these infertility grant opportunities are fairly new. As a result, the overall implementation of these types of programs just isn't up to snuff yet. Overall, we prefer the handful of organizations that charge no fee and have been around for a while. We are still left with more questions than answers at this point. If it fits with your plan, you don't need to rule it out, but buyer beware.

Egg Sharing

"I just participated in the one of the few clinics that does the shared donor egg program. They pair up a woman who has eggs but can't really afford her IVF with someone who needs eggs. I was a donor.

I put a profile in a book and was chosen one month later by a recipient. I had to write a twenty-page term paper on my life and submit childhood photos.

"Once picked, they put me on birth control pills to match our cycles together. Then I got stimulated with the meds and turned into a chicken. I made forty eggs. Talk about discomfort! Then I had the retrieval, which was uneventful. Only thirteen of them matured, and I kept six eggs, and the rest of the mature eggs went to her. It only cost me $4,500 total for my IVF, with nothing covered by insurance. The program recipient paid for my stim meds, egg retrieval, and anesthesia."

—BELLA

I know it's nice to share, but should I really share my eggs? And how? A few IVF clinics have introduced an egg-sharing program whereby patients who cannot afford the cost of IVF treatment receive it in return for donating a percentage of the eggs harvested to matching paying recipients. The recipient pays for most of the donor's treatment, but it is still cheaper than a traditional egg-donor program.

Here's how it works: an infertile woman undergoes IVF treatment. After the eggs are retrieved, they are shared between the infertile couple and the egg recipient couple, with the recipient getting any "odd" number of eggs. The minimum number of eggs for sharing is usually eight, but varies between different centers. Or, depending on the program, the donor has "first pick" of at least four eggs before the rest are given to other women. The donor pays for her own daily labs, ultrasounds, the ICSI, and embryo transfer.

The potential egg sharer donor is carefully assessed and screened for infectious and genetic diseases. Potential donors with known or suspected poor ovarian response or poor egg quality are excluded. The egg sharer donor must be fit and healthy, under the age of thirty-five with an FSH (blood hormone level) of less than 8. She should have no history of ovarian disease or surgery.

Once each woman has her own egg cache, then the eggs are inseminated with their respective partners' sperm. Each couple will have their own embryos transferred. Generally, the process is anonymous, the donor and recipient never meet, and you won't know if pregnancy is achieved in the other woman.

There is some concern that this won't work as well because the donor obviously has impaired fertility or she wouldn't be doing IVF. But initial research looks promising—and there are lots of reasons people need IVF that have nothing to do with egg quality. A study in the *Journal of Human Reproduction* shows egg-sharing programs do not decrease the chance of pregnancy for the egg donor. They effectively decrease wait time for donor eggs and increase funding resources for donors who also require fertility treatment. There are no significant differences in pregnancy rates among the three groups.

And yet, not many clinics do it. Dr. Mark Perloe refuses to do egg-sharing cycles. "Most IVF programs avoid this procedure because of increased stress and concerns if the number of eggs is limited. I believe that the time, stress, and expense associated with assisted reproductive technologies require doing everything possible to ensure the best chance of success. Giving away half your eggs is not, in my opinion, the most cost-effective approach to pregnancy."

It isn't right for everyone. The time and coordination involved are cost-prohibitive for clinics as well. Two women must have their cycles timed very closely. And as with any ART cycle, the donor treatment cycle does not always go as planned. For example, not enough eggs are collected. Just as in a regular egg donation cycle, there is no guarantee of success, even with a proven donor. If the donor is not stimulating well and is not showing at least ten nicely progressing follicles by day seven, the cycle will usually be canceled. The eggs may fail to fertilize or the embryos may not divide.

If you're interested, and your clinic doesn't offer a program, you may want to consider using a private agency to do the matching for you. Agency for Shared Cycle Solutions, Inc., for example, offers a database of potential donors, helps coordinate the cycles with the clinic, and takes care of the legal and psychological details. There are other agencies, and you'll want to compare costs carefully. Factor in costs for travel, as some programs require you to use selected clinics.

SHARING A TRADITIONAL DONOR'S EGGS

Another option is to have a shared, or "split," cycle, in which two couples undergo IVF using the eggs from one anonymous donor. The couples enjoy the combined benefits of having viable eggs toward a healthy pregnancy at half the usual cost of egg donation.

Through such a program, couples pay only half of the usual expenses for the donor's services. Donor-related costs include recruitment and screening expenses, all related monitoring and medical care for the ovulation stimulation and retrieval processes, donor compensation, and insurance. The receiving couples are provided with profiles that include a childhood photo of the donor, a listing of nonidentifying physical characteristics, psychosocial background (such as hobbies, interests, and talents), and medical information and history on all members of the donor's family of origin.

The cycles of each couple are synchronized with the egg donor's cycles. Once the eggs are retrieved, they are shared between the recipients. In a donor egg cycle, an average of 21 eggs are retrieved. Sixty percent (13) of those eggs fertilize and 40 percent (8) of the fertilized eggs produce good quality embryos. One clinic's experience with 800 shared donor egg cycles found:

- In 60 percent of cycles, a single donor makes enough eggs to share with three recipients.
- In 20 percent of cycles, there are enough for two recipients.
- In 10 percent of cycles, there are only enough for one recipient.
- In 10 percent of cycles there is an insufficient number of eggs, and the procedure is canceled.

Again, you may have to do some research to find a clinic willing to consider this option. If coordinating two people's cycles is tricky, working with three is downright difficult.

SHARING WITH YOUR CLINIC

Because some clinics are having success with frozen eggs, they are requesting all egg donor recipients to "contribute" some of the eggs retrieved from their donors to the clinic's egg bank in order to build their supplies. In exchange for a discounted fee, you will be limited in the number of eggs you are allowed to keep and the rest are turned over to the clinic's egg bank.

One such clinic is limiting the number of donor eggs you can keep to 12, with the rest going to the bank. Don't accept this without some tough questions. You bought those eggs. Since there is no way to "grade" the eggs, they are randomly distributed. With enough bad luck, you could be left with the 12 worst eggs of the bunch. And truly, how many of us with infertility consider ourselves lucky? Considering most clinics shoot for 20 to 30 eggs in one cycle, you are getting less than half of the eggs for just a few thousand dollars' discount. It's one thing if it is completely up to whether you want to participate in this or not. But if the clinic tries to force (or even strongly encourages) you to do this, it's not playing fair.

To add insult to injury, the clinics might make recipients eat the costs of donor screening and stimulation while the clinic benefits from the extra eggs. This is going to become more popular among clinics over time as attempts to freeze eggs continue to increase, so ask about these types of split cycles. Don't inadvertently sign with a clinic that forces you to do a split cycle for its fiscal benefit and at greater risk for you. If you are going to pay more than $20,000 for egg donation, you need as many eggs as possible. In our opinion, giving up a lot of eggs to save a few thousand dollars doesn't save enough money to justify the risk.

Sharing with Researchers

Depending on which way political winds blow, using eggs and embryos for research is becoming more common. In July 2006, stem cell researchers were given permission to recruit human egg donors for research using egg-sharing programs. Under this egg-sharing model, the research team contributes to the cost of a patient's IVF treatment in return for the donation of some of her eggs. The material would be used in a field of stem cell research known as nuclear transfer, or therapeutic cloning.

Obviously, egg sharing in any capacity isn't to be done without careful consideration. You'll have to imagine how you will cope if you do not get pregnant and do not have leftover eggs for another cycle. Most clinics have counselors or can refer you to mental health professionals trained in helping couples work through psychological and moral issues. Just because you have a new option to consider doesn't mean it's right for you and your partner.

Too Good to Be True

What's possible in infertility treatment today wasn't even imagined twenty years ago. And a decade from now, the field will look completely different. After all, infertility is big business, and researchers, doctors, and corporations want as much of the pie as they can get their hands on. Egg freezing will undoubtedly become more effective, genetic testing will become increasingly sophisticated, and IVF success rates will climb. Medications, laboratory techniques, and medical procedures continue to improve. One infertility business is generating plenty of controversy, and a few interested investors and clients, by attempting to create an embryo bank. You would be able to purchase embryos they create through the use of sperm and egg donors.

As you check with Dr. Google over every infertility term you can think of and spend hours "net surfing," you'll come across articles and advertisements, even personal testimonials, about the latest, greatest new thing. Be wary. Ovulation watches, $5,000 worth of acupuncture, infertility yoga, and fertility-boosting supplements may be effective only in draining your checkbook. When something seems too good to be true, evaluate the claims for yourself to determine if the treatment would be an appropriate option for you. When looking at a new product, technique, or option, ask yourself these questions:

- Consider the source: Is there legitimate corroboration? Is it from a journal article, physician, friend, or blog?
- Were the people who were successful just like you? Do they even exist?
- Can you afford it?
- Are you willing to go to the time and trouble to do this?
- Can you think of any possible harm if you try this?
- Would it interfere with your current treatments or cause you to have to stop all other treatment to do this?

Personal Fund-Raising

*"It's amazing how many treasures people are willing to part with
when they know the money is going to a good cause: curio cabinets,
dining room sets, televisions, anything you can imagine. After
announcing through an email that we were going to be holding a
yard sale to raise money for our adoption efforts, Mike and I drove
a truck from house to house picking up items from people we knew
and even some people we didn't know who heard of our plans and
wanted to help. We earned nearly $1,000 and we had enough items
left over to do another yard sale."*

JENNA

The key to figure out how to raise money is by appealing to what people love to do: they love to help, and they love to have fun. Those are the perfect ingredients for a good game of Texas Hold 'Em. By inviting a few friends over and providing inexpensive food and beverages, several hundred dollars can be raised before you know it. Imagine that a typical night out with friends might cost around $50. Now imagine hosting a poker night where the ante is $50, but half of the money goes to family-building efforts and the other half goes to the winner. By the end of the night, a financially strapped infertile couple with ten friends could walk away with a few hundred dollars (even more if you win).

Create a Web Page

One couple has received national attention for their cyber-creativity to raise funds for their infertility treatment. Due to male-factor infertility, Shelton and Brandi Koskie learned their best bet was IVF. The problem? They were $15,000 short. The solution? They created Babyorbust.com, an online cyber-begging site to solicit donations to pay for treatment. Several thousand dollars have poured in, but not quite enough to cover their medical expenses.

*"BabyorBust.com was founded on the idea that we could open
people's eyes to IVF and the expense and emotion that it brings
with it. Every doctor's appointment, lab test, poke, prod, and*

Band-aid comes out of our hip pocket. We earn a reasonable salary,
we live a fairly comfortable lifestyle, but we do not have twenty Gs
lying around. That's why we're asking the world to help us out."

—BRANDI KOSKIE

SOLICITING FUNDS ON THE INTERNET

If you use the web to solicit funds, consider adding a tool like the ChipIn widget to your webpage. ChipIn, and its up-and-coming competitors, are simple Flash applications that let your social network contribute via a secure service and collect your funds via PayPal, direct deposit, or check. It can be used on MySpace pages, type pad blogs, and other social networking sites. ChipIn does not charge any fees if you raise less than $10,000.

Fund-Raising Companies

Some companies have targeted fund-raising for those seeking funds for adoption and infertility research and sell products you can resell at a profit. For example, A Child's Desire is a company founded by an adoptive mom who helps families raise money for infertility and adoption expenses. Valerie Gagnon, company founder, represents companies from Avon to the Pampered Chef and Tupperware. "The way it works is simple. You pass the catalogs and fund-raising flyers around to family, friends, coworkers, and neighbors. Anyone can assist you with your fund-raiser. Family and friends can distribute your fund-raiser even if they live in another state. All orders are sent to me for processing. Shortly after your products are delivered, your profit checks are sent under separate cover."

Products run the gamut from coffee to candles to coupon books. Profits vary as well, from 7 percent to 20 percent of total sales, with the remainder of the money going back to the fund-raising company. Do your homework: see how long they've been in business and ask to speak to other customers. The best are those who have a relationship with the Better Business Bureau, which they can join even if they have only an online store. When choosing a direct sales company as a way to raise additional money, think about these factors:

- Choose a product you love, whether it is baskets, candles, or makeup.
- Consider choosing a product you already know something about.
- When researching companies, start with companies you know and like.
- Look at the company's record of accomplishments.
- Go for companies that have been around a while and have good track records.
- Ask about the required investment, your commission, and sales requirements.

You may find raising money for adoption to be easier than raising money for infertility. However unfair, adoption seems more like a "sure thing" than infertility treatments to many people.

Change Jobs or Move for Better Insurance

What if your health insurance is the pits and your HR department can't be swayed? Consider a job change—or even a move to a fertility-friendly state. Research companies with great IVF insurance, and if you have a fairly portable job, like nursing, make a switch. If the coverage is substantially better, it might even be worth a pay cut. Some companies offer health insurance for part-time employees, usually beginning at twenty hours a week. You may even find a company with infertility benefits is more family friendly

---

QUESTIONS TO CONSIDER ABOUT HEALTH INSURANCE

- If you are married, is your spouse covered?
- If you are not married and want to cover your partner, will your health insurance plan cover him or her?
- Are the available insurance programs what you need?
- How is infertility covered?
- Are there adoption benefits?

and better to work for in the long run. *Conceive* and *Working Mother* magazines regularly publish lists of the best companies to work for in regards to infertility and adoption coverage.

Wait until you have a job offer to discuss employee benefits, either with the human resources department or with the person who is offering you the job. Request a copy of the current health insurance policy. It is much better to be fully informed before you accept a position than it is to have an unpleasant surprise later on.

> *"Infertility has taken a lot out of us, but it hasn't drained all of our resources. We still have our ingenuity and determination. As long as we have that, we'll be able to find our way to the money that will help us buy happiness."*
>
> —Sally

Five Things You Can Do Right Now

1. Bookmark clinicaltrials.gov and start checking every week to see if you qualify for any trials.
2. Check current IVF grant requirements and see if you qualify. If so, start writing.
3. Determine if your clinic participates in any clinical trials.
4. Ask your clinic about options like egg sharing if you are interested.
5. Consider if any other options, such as creating a personal fundraising page, would be appropriate for your situation.

CHAPTER 11

Broaden Your Horizons:
Travel for Treatment

"I remember flying interstate for my frozen embryo transfer and at the time I felt like I was on a top-secret mission involving the couriering of a special package. That the package happened to be in my womb didn't matter, it still felt as if there should be some kind of protocol surrounding it—an embryo-guard escort, for instance.

"But should you fly when undergoing IVF? Probably not if you have a crippling fear of flying and require heavy sedation before the plane leaves the aerobridge."

—JODI PANAYOTOV, author of the book
In Vitro Fertility Goddess

WHAT IF THE BEST CARE for you isn't in your own backyard? What if you don't live close to any fertility specialists? Or what if the only one you're close to isn't the right fit? You may save money by leaving town for another fertility clinic if the prices are substantially different. Your options are only as limited to how far you're willing to travel.

Closer to Home

"For me, traveling to another state was totally worth it. I had all the blood work done at my doctor's office the first cycle. Then I had all my blood work done at a lab the second/frozen transfer and that was easier. The drive wasn't bad either, and we rested the day before the transfer and a day after. We are going to do it again in the next year or two."

—ANNA

Clinics in the same geographical area typically charge very similar fees. To get a considerable price cut for the same chance at success, you might have to leave the area. Traveling even one hundred miles can save 30 percent or more on treatment fees. Prices for one IVF can vary significantly in different parts of the country. For example, one clinic's fee for egg retrieval and embryo transfer is only $3,500. But just two hours away, another clinic charges almost double that. And if you go another four hours, the price is substantially higher at $8,300.

There are not-so-subtle pressures placed on doctors who charge substantially lower fees. "I have received complaints from more than one physician for not charging my patients more. I'd rather charge the lowest amount I can, without turning anybody away, and I'll match my success rates up against anybody," says one lower-cost fertility specialist.

If you need an egg donor, traveling might be the best way to save money. Donor compensation varies from state to state. Some areas average fees around $2,000, while generally, more metropolitan areas are quadruple that amount. As a rule, though, everywhere in the Northeast and the West Coast is expensive. Some states, like Indiana and Utah, have laws restricting donor egg compensation to less than $3,000. You might be placed on a waiting list, but if it works, you've saved about 40 percent to 60 percent. Questions to consider about traveling for fertility treatments:

- Do you have any frequent flier miles just waiting to be used?
- Where do your far-flung friends and family members live? Not having to pay for accommodations saves big bucks.
- If your insurance covers at least a portion of the cost, what limitations are there to leaving the area?
- Will your insurance company reimburse you for out-of-pocket travel costs if you can prove you do not have local access to care? Some do.

Compare success rates and prices—traveling for a better price is no bargain if you cut your odds of having a baby. Start a list of some of the centers you would consider going to. Maybe you go to certain cities frequently or you have family or friends there. Start with our "State by State" guide in the appendices and consider if any other locales would be a better option.

If you are considering traveling within the United States to see a fertility specialist, call the office to ask your basic questions about the practice.

- Set up a consultation with the physician via phone or email.
- Complete the office's patient history form and return it for the doctor to review before consult.
- Send copies of relevant diagnostic workups and treatments.
- Find a local physician to coordinate the ultrasounds and monitoring during the stimulation phase. Some clinics have relationships with other fertility specialists throughout the country who can help with this.
- Plan your trip for egg retrieval and embryo transfer.

Going Abroad

"Going to India for IVF was the best decision we ever made. The complete cost for donor eggs, medications, lab, and medical costs was only $5,000. It cost another $5,000 for airfare, food, and hotel, but it was still cheaper than the fertility clinic in my city. I saved over $5,000 doing this. We only had $10,000 to work with. It was this or nothing. It would have been more convenient to be closer to home, but it simply wasn't an option for us."

—PAULETTE

Do people really do it? Do they really get passports, wave good-bye to the familiar faces at their local fertility clinic, and take off to fertility specialists unknown? There are fertility clinics in at least twenty-eight countries on four continents that cater to the international health traveler. The single biggest reason Americans travel to other countries for infertility treatment is to save money. Depending upon the country and what exactly you need, you can reasonably expect 15 percent to 85 percent savings over the cost of treatment in the United States. Or, as one infertility patient explained, "I took out my credit card instead of a second mortgage on my home."

The vast majority of Americans who are infertile look for help close to home. A small number, though—no one keeps an official count—are seek-

POPULAR DESTINATIONS FOR IVF*

1. India
2. South Korea
3. Czech Republic
4. Barbados
5. Greece
6. Colombia
7. South Africa
8. Mexico
9. New Zealand
10. Spain

*Several of the countries do not allow donor eggs or donor sperm.

ing help in places such as South Africa, Israel, Italy, Germany, Sweden, the Czech Republic, and Singapore, where costs can be much lower.

Dr. Aniruddha Malpani, author of *How to Have a Baby: A Guide for the Infertile Couple* and director of the Malpani Infertility Clinic in Bombay, India, has been practicing IVF for fifteen years. "In the last two, three years, we have treated many couples who come from the US and the UK. In fact, the majority of our patients these days come from abroad. Medical tourists can be demanding patients! They have lost faith in their own medical system; and many of them are doctors and nurses who make their own medical decisions. They are challenging to treat, and I enjoy doing so, because they are well-informed and capable of thinking out of the box—it does take guts to travel to India for medical treatment! We go out of our way to build a world-class reputation by being transparent, accountable, responsive, and patient-centric."

Besides cost savings, many report receiving better quality care. According to Josef Woodman, author of *Patients Beyond Borders: Everybody's Guide to Affordable, World-Class Medical Tourism*, foreign clinics boast VIP waiting lounges, deluxe hospital suites, and staffed recuperation resorts, along with free transportation to and from airports, low-cost meal plans for companions, and discounted hotels affiliated with the hospital.

Infertility Treatment Costs by Country

SERVICE	BARBADOS	CZECH REPUBLIC	INDIA
IVF	$6,000	$2,925	$2,500
IVF with Donor Eggs	$8,500	$4,350	$5,000

Magdalena Cogbill, founder of My IVF Alternative, which helps people seek lower-cost infertility treatments in the Czech Republic, reports her clients are always impressed with the state-of-the-art facilities as well as the quality of the physicians, most of whom were trained in the United States or Europe. "Patients receive a lot more personal attention in the Czech Republic than in the United States," explains Cogbill, who lives in the United States half of the year. "Great lengths are taken to ensure clients are well taken care of before, during, and after their treatments."

Anna Hosford, clinical director at Barbados Fertility Centre, explains, "We would never pretend going through an IVF program would not be stressful. But with a number of recent studies, psychologists have established that by reducing stress levels during fertility treatments, a marked increase of a successful outcome is achieved. With that knowledge, what better place in the world to reduce your stress than on the exotic island of Barbados in the Caribbean?"

Anne, who traveled to Sweden for IVF, was shocked to find she had continual access to her doctor via his cell phone. "It's a different system. I would never in a million years have been given my fertility specialist's cell phone number back home. At home, if I had a question, I'd leave a message on the clinic answering machine and then a nurse would call me back. If she didn't know the answer and needed to ask the doctor, she'd call him and then call me back again. We could play phone tag all day while I was at work trying to whisper so no one would know what I was doing."

Preliminary reports suggest that, if chosen carefully, the best international clinics offer success rates comparable to those of the best clinics in the United States. There are no studies that compare success rates internationally, so you'll have to do your homework and plenty of it.

The service may be better, the cost will almost certainly be lower, and you'll have an opportunity to spend a few weeks away from "normal" life with its stresses and hectic pace. One of the advantages of leaving town for IVF is that you're forced to be away from work and other typical responsibilities. You can relax, sightsee as you're interested, and maybe even reconnect with your partner.

Want to plan how long you will need to be gone? Check out the IVF treatment calendar at http://www.drmalpani.com/ivfcalendar.htm.

Is it really safe? After all, nobody wants to end up trusting their precious eggs to a quack in a shack. Or pay thousands to be treated in a clinic where the embryology lab is suspect. Don't book the first clinic that comes up in a web search. Nothing is that easy in infertility. Research your options carefully. Once you've chosen at least half a dozen, narrow your options based on your travel preferences, geography, budget, time requirements, and other variables. Consider these factors:

- **Check accreditation.** Some hospitals offer fertility services that are Joint Commission accredited. While it isn't essential for hospitals, the Joint Commission is the only American seal of approval that shows that a hospital meets a superior standard of care. The accreditation process is rigorous, and you can feel more confident in a hospital willing to do the legwork required for such a process. Other hospitals may not be Joint Commission approved but may have local accreditation.

- **Look for partnerships between overseas hospitals and American medical centers.** Johns Hopkins, Duke, and Harvard are all involved in international medical care, and those affiliations may provide you with an extra level of comfort. Also, reputable clinics outside the United States should have some type of affiliation with the American Society for Reproductive Medicine (ASRM) or the European Society for Human Reproduction and Embryology (ESHRE) to ensure they are abiding by strict ethical standards and guidelines set forth by their peers.

- **Research the licensing requirements in the country you are considering.** For example, laboratories that deal with human tissue (like embryology labs) may need to be regulated. Find out what the licensing body is and confirm each clinic's accreditation with the licensing agency, not with the clinic itself.

- **Ask for the physician's résumé.** Check it out. Talk to at least five professional references. Many fertility specialists are trained in the United States or Britain, and you may find that to be reassuring as well.

- **Ask for contact information from former patients, especially someone who was not successful.** Talk to at least five patients. While getting names from the clinic is one way, you won't get unbiased patients. Seek out online forums and find patients there. Ask lots of questions. What did they wish they had known? Would they do it again?

- **Check out the media locally.** Has a clinic been featured in the local media? If so, that can be a good sign, but get the article translated to confirm what it says.

- **Ask if you can speak to the doctor personally about your case on the phone before you book your trip.** Does the medical team speak English fluently? Infertility is a complicated issue and you must be able to communicate effectively with the medical staff to ensure good quality care.

- **Get everything in writing so you can compare clinics' costs carefully.** Makes sure you're comparing apples and apples. What exactly does the IVF fee cover? Does it include medications? Are there hidden extras like blood work, anesthesia, or ultrasounds?

- **Expect to see success rates.** All of them. They should be broken down by age and procedure. The success rate of thirty-year-olds isn't relevant to you if you're forty. Find out if they select only certain kinds of patients to keep their success rates high. In other words, do they turn away women older than thirty-five?

- **Know what you need.** Don't go until you have had a thorough workup—and a second opinion. If you have had three failed IVF cycles already and your fertility specialist suggests donor eggs, getting the same IVF treatment in another country isn't a good use of your resources.

- **Trust your instincts.** There isn't one right answer. Traveling isn't the right answer for everyone. If you decide to go, there will be at least one person in your life who thinks it's a bad idea. There's no perfect clinic, either here or internationally. Several clinics could be really good choices for you, so do your homework, but trust your gut. Hop on the next flight back home if it doesn't feel right.

Before You Book that Flight

"Something else that factored into my initial research—though only in terms of additional advantages and not as a way to rule various clinics out—was the geographical location of the clinic. For instance, I'd always wanted to visit Ireland, so I checked to see whether or not it would be possible to undergo egg donation procedures in Ireland. It wasn't. We checked to see whether or not it was possible to have the procedure performed in the Scandinavian country where my friend was living, but egg donation isn't allowed there—only sperm donation. We also preferred not to go anywhere that would necessitate making complex travel plans, having to change flights, or requiring extensive land travel after the flight. It was fascinating to discover which countries allowed egg donation and which did not, as well as the degree of industry regulation in each country—some countries adhere to more strict regulations, while others seem to maintain more of a 'wild west' attitude.

"Some of the less expensive clinics in parts of Eastern Europe targeted Americans and other Westerners, luring them with complete travel packages, touring during the stay, assistance with ground logistics, et cetera. The clinic we used in Spain had a branch in Valencia that included an international department, which could arrange, among other things, foreign language speakers speaking a variety of languages. We used the branch in Madrid because a friend had recommended it and because it was more convenient, but it was sometimes difficult to break through the language barrier, as many of the Spaniards we encountered, though friendly and helpful, didn't know English very well, and I imagine that this could be an issue with a number of clinics in non-English-speaking countries as well."

—Eliza

You may want to look for a health travel planner, suggests Josef Woodman. A qualified agent is usually a specialist in a given region or treatment, with the best doctors, accommodations, and in-country contacts at her fingertips. Once you've settled on your health travel destination, it pays to seek out the services of that locale's best health travel agent. Agents usually pay for themselves and are well worth the relatively modest additional fees they typically charge. They should know plenty about your destination's current and upcoming public health concerns as well.

If you have any insurance coverage, it's not going to pay for anything out of the country. You also have to decide what you can live with. If you don't conceive after traveling for an IVF cycle, would you regret having gone and wish you had saved your money toward a cycle at home?

What Does a Health Travel Planner Do?

- Matches patients with the appropriate physicians;
- Supplies data on hospital accreditations, physician's credentials, board affiliations, number of surgeries performed, association memberships, and ongoing training;
- Arranges telephone consultations between patients and doctors;
- Handles travel arrangements, including obtaining visas and reserving lodging;
- Expedites transfer of patient's medical information;
- Plans leisure activities;
- Provides use of an international cell phone;
- Arranges translators and accompaniment to medical appointments;
- Assists with any difficulties experienced when you get home with paperwork, records, or prescriptions.

International Egg Donors

"Kathryn Butuceanu longed for children. But at her age, her best hope lay in fertility clinics and an egg donor, a quest she soon found could easily cost up to $72,000 for repeated tries.... Help came through a call to Dr. Sanford Rosenberg, a fertility specialist in Richmond, Virginia, who started a program capitalizing on lower medical costs overseas. By using an egg donor from Romania, having the eggs fertilized in Bucharest and then shipped back to the United States, the Butuceanus cut their costs to $18,000, including enough fertilized eggs for repeated efforts."*

Perhaps the biggest way to save money overseas is by using third-party donors in other countries. Again, you'll need to research this well because you're adding another level of complexity, but it can be done. Or, you can stay home, like the Butuceanus. You will need to ship your sperm over in order for the fertility clinic to fertilize the eggs. Once fertilization takes place, the embryos are frozen and shipped back to you in care of your state-side fertility clinic.

Egg donation is much cheaper in other countries. In India, for example, you pay the clinic only $1,000 for an egg donor. Of course, depending on the country, you may have limited options for selection. Don't expect any blond, blue-eyed donors in India or Barbados. Prices vary substantially, depending on the country, and there are countries that do not allow egg donation or compensation for egg donors, so eggs are in limited supply.

Ideally, the donor should be a nonsmoking woman less who is younger than thirty years old, has no history of prior infertility herself, is of normal body weight, and has an unremarkable medical and genetic history. There are no international guidelines for regulating egg donation, and that raises ethical concerns. In developing countries there is enormous opportunity for poorer women to be exploited when money becomes the primary motivation for donating eggs or undergoing surrogacy procedures. Find out how much donors are paid and how much the center profits from the donor egg fee. How are donors informed of the risks of the process? Consider the significant amount of time, risk, and medical intervention she is going through to provide you with eggs.

As much as you want to get pregnant, you don't want to live with a guilty conscience, either. It isn't right to pay a poor woman in a third world country only $100 for her eggs, regardless of how much that $100 would buy in her economy. You want your process to have integrity, so you know your donor was treated in an ethical and humane manner. Remember, how they treat their donors may indicate how they treat their recipients as well.

---

*Felicia R. Lee, "Driven by Costs, Fertility Clients Head Overseas," *New York Times*, January 25, 2005.

International Surrogacy

"I am having a woman from India carry our baby. I cannot conceive on my own. My clinic actually has nutritionists and nurses visit the surrogate moms so they get all they need health-wise. I am grateful to all these people and especially to the surrogate mom for doing for me what I could not do for myself."

—Lucy

If surrogacy is your only option, it is possible to arrange it in another country. Compared to the $60,000 to $100,000 for surrogacy in the United States, you may be able to have an international surrogate for around $25,000.

INTERNATIONAL SURROGACY FEES FOR INDIA*

The average cost is $25,000, and the fees are divided into four stages:

Stage 1: $4,000
Recruiting, preparing, screening surrogate
IVF fees
Transportation and accommodations for surrogate

Stage 2: $4,000
Egg donor fees or meds and retrieval for intended mom
Travel costs for ten days for intended parents

Stage 3: Confirmation of pregnancy, $13,000
Pregnancy care
Delivery fee
Surrogate fee (approximately $7,000)

Stage 4: $3,000
Legal fees
Documentation costs for baby
Travel costs for intended parents to bring home baby

*Sample fees from Planet Hospital.

To date, India is the most popular locale for surrogates, but the possibility exists that other countries will jump on the bandwagon since profit is involved.

One big caveat: You have little recourse legally if something goes wrong in the process. Again, you'll need to consider carefully what fees would be just for what you are asking another person to do. You have no guarantee about how your surrogate is being treated. In India, some agencies use homes for surrogate mothers, which isolate women from their own families during the process. Some women keep this a secret and say they are working in another city and cannot see their own children during the pregnancy.

International surrogacy raises the same concerns as egg donation and others, too. After all, the risks of pregnancy and childbirth can be far greater in another country compared to in the United States. You will also have less contact with the surrogate mom compared to the relationships that might develop in the United States. Ideally, you would spend a month with her during the egg retrieval and embryo transfer, and you spend time with her again during delivery. Because of the distance and language barrier, you will not get to know her or truly know how she is doing. While this might be worth considering if you feel you have no other options, it is far from ideal for anyone involved.

Different Treatment Options

When you travel to other countries, you have access to different treatment options than in the United States. Whether that's a good thing depends on who you ask. Some procedures may not be done yet in the States because they haven't been tested enough; others may have been done previously but are no longer permitted or regularly practiced. Cytoplasmic transfer, for example, where cytoplasm from a healthy donor egg is implanted into a patient's weaker egg, is illegal here but still an option in other countries.

> *"Cytoplasmic transfer totally worked for me. And that's why I'm such an advocate for it, because I tried four in vitros, and nothing worked. My eggs weren't of good quality. So I figured, why not try this, add a little protein, make it a healthier, stronger egg? And sure*

enough, it did work for me. But doctors said she's gonna have chromosomal abnormalities, so I did have that tested, and she's fine. She's totally healthy."

—Sharon, who had the procedure done in Lebanon

Nuclear transfer is also banned in the United States. Similar to the above process, nuclear transfers result in eggs that have the female donor's cytoplasm—and the mother's nucleus, which houses the genes for everything from hair color to height. Another treatment not regularly practiced here now but found in some European clinics is lymphocyte immune therapy for women with recurrent spontaneous abortions. This therapy uses blood products from others to prompt the patient's own immune system to recognize the pregnancy.

Another difference in treatment beyond some country's borders is the number of transferred embryos. Once you've got them, how many will you throw back in? In current fertility center practices, two embryos is the norm, and only very rarely will physicians transfer more than three. Women will usually have to have had at least one failed IVF and be over forty to even consider having three embryos implanted. The emphasis is instead on transferring only the best embryos that have the greatest chance of success. Multiple births, especially higher than twins, are not considered successful in most U.S. clinics today. But that does not mean you won't find clinics all over the world that suggest otherwise.

India allows six embryos at a time. The risk, of course, is a higher-order multiple pregnancy, which has extraordinary risks for mom and babies. Paulette, who gave birth to a healthy son after IVF in India, had six embryos implanted. "I knew it was a risk I was taking. But it felt like the right thing to do." While Paulette was lucky to have just one healthy baby, you need to know the risks related to transferring multiple embryos. If selective reduction is not a procedure you would consider, carefully weigh your options regarding the number of embryos implanted.

Travel Tips for Traveling Abroad for Infertility Treatments

- **Plan ahead.** If you are considering traveling out of the country, renew or apply for your passport soon, as delays can sometimes take months.

- **Consider your transportation.** If there are fertility clinics within a five- to six-hour drive, you may decide to drive instead of fly. If you're going solo for at least one way, decide how far you feel comfortable driving.
- **Invest in the right ticket.** Airline tickets can be pricey and may eat up a significant portion of your costs if you are looking at traveling either domestically or abroad. No bargain-basement airline tickets here. Do not buy fourteen-day advance-purchase tickets; you need open-ended tickets. As you know, with infertility, anything can happen. If you don't respond to the protocol, you will want to cancel the cycle and reschedule. Don't take a chance of losing your ticket by saving money. It's too much of a gamble.

Coordinating with Your Home Physician

Once you decide to travel more than a few hours away, you still need to have a physician you feel comfortable with close to home. You are going to need help with pretreatment tests, getting your records together, preparing for travel, and after-treatment follow-up care.

Whether you are traveling near or far, you must have a local physician to do blood work and ultrasound monitoring as well as other follow-up care. The blood work can be done at any lab, but finding someone to do your ultrasounds is important. In addition, you'll want to have an established relationship with a health care professional if complications arise before and after treatment.

"I have not had any problems with women finding physicians willing to do their monitoring before traveling to my office," says Dr. James Donahue. "I prefer for a fertility specialist's office to do the monitoring for two reasons. First, we speak the same language and have similar enough training that I can feel confident in what they are reporting. Second, they are almost always open on weekends, which many gynecologist offices are not."

Medications

If you are traveling within the United States, you will need to find a pharmacy that will accept your prescription (particularly if it is in a different state) or you will need to bring your medications with you. If your fertility drugs need to be refrigerated, you'll need to find a way to keep them cold. You have a couple of options. They now sell a portable fridge you can put in your car for a drive and then move into wherever you are staying. You can also try to find a hotel with a fridge in the room. For short trips by car, or until you get to the hotel, you can purchase a diabetic care kit for traveling with your medications; these usually have a case, needles, portable needle disposal or sharps case, and a way to refrigerate the medication.

If you are traveling internationally, be careful, since some medications cannot be taken across national borders, and some medications may not be available in all countries. You may need a prescription to carry syringes or medications on board an airplane as well. Most likely, your medications can be purchased in the country where you are having the treatment, resulting in additional cost savings since pharmaceutical prices are lower overseas. These are all important details you will want to have clearly defined before you pack your bags. If you are entering a different time zone, keep your watch on your time zone. This prevents you from having to do the math to take your medications.

Should I or Shouldn't I?

Ideally, we would love to say you could get the best, most cost-effective treatment close to home. There is no doubt infertility treatment is expensive and out of the reach of most. If you've exhausted all your other options, and traveling to achieve your dream of having a baby is all you have left, you'll need to follow careful guidelines, take precautions, and do your research to guarantee you are getting the best care. "Good planning is essential to the success of any medical procedure, and that goes double for the global patient," says Josef Woodman. "But with diligence, perseverance, and good information, traveling abroad for treatment is a legitimate, affordable and safe choice."

Five Things You Can Do Right Now
1. Consider if traveling outside your hometown is an option for you.
2. Research three clinics in the United States you might consider.

3. Research three clinics outside the United States you might consider.
4. Look on online forums to find people who have gone to the clinics you are considering.
5. If an international destination is a possibility, ask for recommendations for a health travel planner.

CHAPTER 12

Don't End Up Broke:
Understand Your Financing Options

"I felt in total control of our future . . . but then infertility became part of the picture. We eventually had to take a credit card cash advance for the procedure. It made me cringe as I called the credit card company for the money. What could I do? It's extremely difficult for me not to get angry when I talk about this topic. My financial goals were put on hold indefinitely. My Excel spreadsheet was showing zeros in the additional principal column. I was paying interest on credit card balances because I couldn't afford to pay them off.

"Fear started to set in on how many cycles we could afford to do IVF. We talked about the possibility of selling our house and downsizing our cars to free up additional cash each month. We felt guilty when we ordered out and became increasing more aware of unnecessary lights that were on in the house. We had to save all our money to combat the infertility demon. I was also getting depressed because I knew once we had children it would be a long road just to pay off the current debt. Plans of Jenna taking time off to care for the baby were distant memories.

"I started to become jealous of my married friends. They were all taking their noninfertility money and putting it toward other things, like house improvements, dining room sets, and increasing their retirement contributions. Jenna and I kept taking steps backwards."

—MIKE

MOST CLINICS REQUIRE THAT YOU pay for treatments up front before you can start. Whether it is $2,000, $20,000, $60,000, $100,000, or more, it is difficult to come up with this money in cash at a moment's notice. As a result, it is nearly impossible to come out of infertility treatment without at least some debt.

As you start down the path toward parenthood, it's crucial to find a plan that fits with your wallet. The good news is that there are financing options that allow you to become pregnant and still have money left over for your children. Don't let lack of money or bad insurance coverage stand in the way of your dreams of having children.

Too Much Debt

"We completed two rounds of IVF. The first round was unsuccessful and left us with no leftover embryos. The second round worked and we conceived twins. They were born in October. At the time of IVF my husband worked full-time at a minimum-wage job. I was a first-year teacher. Our total gross income was around $40,000. We took out four loans to pay for our IVF. My mom helped us get the first three loans, and the fourth was through my education credit union. We will be finished paying off our monthly 'baby payment' next summer. We are currently looking at financing IVF with our frozen embryos in an effort to add to our family."

—Amy

With the sky-high costs of infertility treatment, it is tempting to create too much debt with credit cards and loans. Sometimes it's easy to get credit, but it's tough to pay back those debts. Unfortunately, people realize this much too late. Although it takes some organization and advance planning to keep yourself out of debt, it is a lot less work than it takes to dig yourself out of a deep debt hole later.

The most important thing you can do is to keep good records of all your finances—including how much money you have coming in and going out. If you spend more than you earn, you must get it under control if building your family is truly what you want to pursue. It is easy to ignore the spending and hope it will all work out. It won't.

Debt is relative. With infertility, a little debt is practically unavoidable. But a little debt is different from insurmountable debt. People are at different financial stages, so some people have more resources to work with than others. Let's look at some opportunities that help level the playing field.

Special Deals: Multicycle Pricing and Refunds

"A 100 percent refund for IVF if you don't get pregnant" or "A live baby or your money back." The ads are popping up all over the place, but are they for real? For a fixed fee, you have a certain number of chances to overcome your infertility through IVF with a "guarantee" that some portion of the fee will be refunded if you aren't successful. These programs are designed specifically for people who do not have any insurance coverage for infertility. If your insurance company pays for a even little bit of your infertility treatments, you won't qualify.

But what does this mean exactly? And is it a good deal for the rest of us? Basically, in these "risk-sharing," "money-back guarantee," or "multiple-treatment package" plans, the fertility clinic assumes some of the risk for treatment and banks on its ability to achieve conception. Clinics provide a fixed-rate payment plan to cover a specific number of cycles at a discounted fee, with refunds of program fees if conception is not successful after the cycles.

If all cycles are used and produce a baby, the couple receives the cycles at a discounted price. If conception occurs before the completion of all the cycles, the clinic keeps all the money. This structure provides a discount in treatment if it takes several cycles to have a baby and a bonus to the clinic for early success, which is an incentive to the clinic. However, it may create a conflict of interest, causing clinics to take risks they normally wouldn't to get you pregnant quicker. For example, they may encourage you to be more aggressive in the ovulation induction, putting you at risk for ovarian hyperstimulation. After all, the faster you get pregnant, the more money the clinic makes.

> *"The lump sum was big—the cost of a new car—and our fertility specialist did not take a payment plan, so we had to pay for the entire amount up front. But we got our big fat positive on the pregnancy test on our first IVF cycle, and some insensitive person said to me, So since you paid for six cycles, you overpaid for this*

baby then, right? No matter what sacrifices we made for this
pregnancy, we would do it all over again, not just for the positive
pregnancy test but for the peace of mind that came with knowing
that if we didn't get it right on the first try, we could go back to the
drawing board another five times and get our money back if we
weren't able to get pregnant."

—Mandy

Even if different clinics call the program by the same name, the specifics of these types of program vary widely. In price alone these programs can vary anywhere from about $10,000 to $30,000. And number of attempts allowed differs as well as does the actual amount refunded. Some clinics allow six chances, while others allow only three. And some clinics offer a 100 percent money-back guarantee while others refund only 70 percent.

"I almost signed up with a multiple-treatment plan, but once I
looked really closely at everything, I decided it was a pretty big
rip-off. I was quoted three cycles for $30,000 and they claimed
a 100 percent refund, but I had to pay an additional, non-
refundable 20 percent ($6,000) to get the refund. The financial
coordinator called the $6,000 an insurance policy to get the 100
percent refund. If you ask me, that's more like an 83 percent refund
on a $36,000 package. I looked around until I found a better deal."

—Cindy

You better believe they aren't letting just anybody do this deal. They severely limit who can play in this game. After all, they lose money if it doesn't work. The younger you are (typically under thirty-five), the less you will have to pay in terms of a fixed price. Not surprisingly, these costs rise as your age rises. Also, programs penalize women who have gone through previous unsuccessful attempts at IVF. The more unsuccessful attempts you have had, the more you'll have to pay. Having any of the following conditions might also disqualify you from these types of programs:

- more than three unsuccessful attempts;
- being a smoker;
- overweight, or high BMI;

- high FSH levels;
- a history of miscarriages;
- partner with a low sperm count.

And the price doesn't cover everything. Clinics also offer certain "add-ons" in an à la carte fashion for an additional cost as well, including donor eggs, donor sperm, and ultrasound and blood monitoring, PGD, ICSI, and embryo freezing.

Questions to Ask about Money-Back Guarantees or Multiple-Treatment Plan Programs

- What about diagnostics, testing, or prescreening costs?
- How do canceled cycles count toward the number of allowed attempts?
- How many embryos will be transferred?
- Do you have any say as to certain treatment options or decisions?
- What if you are not happy and want to switch clinics?
- What if the clinic wants to terminate us for some reason?
- What if you need to take a break during the treatment?
- What else does this fee cover or *not* cover (i.e., ICSI, cryopreservation, donor sperm, or donor eggs)?

Medication costs, which can run anywhere from $3,000 to $5,000 or more, depending on the particular medication chosen, the dose, and the duration of stimulation needed to get your ovaries to produce as many eggs as possible, are also not included. Because infertility treatments are so individualized, most clinics provide very little information about which end of the range you can expect. Sometimes clinics will cut you a special deal on medications for participating in their multiple-treatment plan package. Even in the best-case scenario, expect to pay a few thousand dollars for medications per each cycle.

Again, what about the statistics? Some programs tout high success rates, including one that claims that 75 percent of patients who complete their infertility treatment refund program for IVF take a baby home. But if the program is so restricted that only the "best" patients get in, how helpful are the success rates?

According to David Schmittlein and Donald Morrison, authors of the article *"A Live Baby or Your Money Back: The Marketing of In Vitro Fertilization Procedures,"* these programs can be profitable only if they involve forceful advertising for more fertile patients, highly selective screening, and aggressive treatment with more side effects and a higher probability of multiple births.

What's the bottom line? While fertility clinics don't like the terminology, this is clearly a marketing strategy. For those of you who fall into the "higher success" category of being under thirty-five and in good health with no previous nonsuccessful attempts at IVF, check to see if your clinic offers this plan. Crunch some numbers and see if this might save you some money overall as opposed to paying for a couple of cycles separately. But know the risks. Read the fine print and ask lots of questions about exactly what is covered and any other additional costs that may be incurred.

> *"We decided to invest in the IVF refund program that our fertility center offers. We just took out a home equity loan for $15,000 and we had $5,000 in savings that we were able to use to pay for the IVF refund program. The program guarantees a baby at the end of two years and six IVFs—all frozen transfers too—or you get all of your $20,000 back. We just finished up IVF number one without success and will be doing our first frozen embryo transfer in the next week or so. Given the disappointment of a negative was hard . . . but not as hard as knowing that we just lost another $10,000. With this program there appears to be light at the end of the tunnel. Even if at the end of two years and six IVFs, we do not have another child, at least we have the money to put toward adoption or a different plan of action."*
>
> —Amberleigh

Clinic Financing

In addition to providing financial counseling to patients, some clinics offer financing programs for infertility treatments. Fertility clinics might allow you to spread out your payments at a set interest rate with a low monthly payment and no prepayment penalties. Many clinics have programs that allow you to plan your payments according to the procedure you have chosen. Ask about up-front or cash payment discounts.

As with any situation in which someone is trying to get you to buy something, don't be pressured into agreeing to terms that you make you feel uncomfortable. Some clinics use slick payment plans to lure you in. Don't be oversold or commit to a finance plan that will leave you scrambling month-to-month. You need to know what you can afford and stick to it. The clinic's finance staff, no matter how nice and helpful they seem, are still working for the clinic. The clinic is their primary responsibility. To ensure a healthy profit margin, they need to convince you to pay as much as possible. If the sales pressure feels too heavy, walk away. Don't sign a payment plan at your first meeting. Take your time and bring a copy home with you.

Paying in Cash

In order to encourage you to pay cash up front, some clinics will offer you a 5 percent to 10 percent discount for doing so. Clinics view this as a benefit because the quicker they can get hold of your money, the quicker they can deposit it into their bank accounts, where it can start earning interest. While this is a big chunk of change for you to part with so quickly, it might be worth your while if you have the cash readily available. Even if your clinic doesn't advertise this type of discount, ask them if they would consider it. On a $20,000 bill, this equates to $1,000 to $2,000 worth of savings.

Third-Party Loans

Since IVF and other infertility treatments can easily add up into the tens of thousands of dollars, taking out a loan might be a necessary evil. There are a few companies out there specializing in financing infertility treatments. These companies have responded to the growing infertility treatment market and cater only to persons undergoing infertility treatments. A benefit of these programs is that you are able to get a loan at a lower interest rate than traditional personal loans or credit cards. Additionally, you don't need to worry about coming up with collateral.

Just like a car loan or mortgage, an unsecured loan requires monthly payments based on a fixed rate and term schedule. The most prominent third-party loan program for infertility treatment is run by Capital One under its health care financing department. They offer fixed rates beginning at 1.99 percent APR (but these go up to 23 percent depending on your credit history), low monthly payments that never change, terms from eighteen to sixty months, and no prepayment penalty. It is the largest patient financing company in the country, but your doctor has to be in the Capital One network for you to qualify. To find out, check with your clinic. If he isn't, your clinic probably works with another financing company. Also, check with your own bank to see if it has any similar programs.

> *"We used Capital One's Healthcare Financing. On this plan, Capital One cuts you a check to pay the doctor, and then you make payments on the loan, just like you'd make a car payment. Our first monthly payment wasn't due until four weeks from the date they received my signed contract. It was easy to apply online, and the interest rates were competitive."*
>
> —SHERI

Assuming you have good credit, these types of loans can be approved within hours. You can borrow anywhere between $1,500 and $25,000 to help pay for infertility treatments. While this may be a good start in getting some cash quick, you can see that even $25,000 won't go very far in paying for infertility treatments. And these loans are not any easier to obtain than they would be from your local bank. You still need a good credit score or your options are limited.

WHAT IS A CREDIT SCORE?

Credit scores usually range from 340 to 850. The higher your score, the less risk the lender believes you will be. As your score climbs, the interest rate you are offered will decline. Borrowers with a credit score of above 700 are typically offered more financing options and better interest rates.

To get a copy of your credit report contact:

Equifax: www.equifax.com
Experian: www.experian.com
Trans Union: www.transunion.com

What if your credit is shaky? You might not be completely out of luck, but you will have fewer options. To get financing, you will definitely pay a higher rate. If you have declared bankruptcy, then you will need a cosigner and it will need to be at least two years since you filed.

Don't saddle yourself with a loan that forces you to borrow more money to pay your monthly bills. The amount you have left over after the bills is the amount you have available for a loan. It is always best to overestimate your expenditures and try to include extra money for those unforeseen expenses that come along. This will help you decide what your loan price range is. Try to avoid longer loans. If the loan is for sixty months, that is five years' worth of interest you are paying in addition to the loan amount.

Loans and Gifts from Friends and Family

"I couldn't believe how expensive an IVF procedure was. There was a stretch of about two months where a day wouldn't go by without receiving a medical bill in the mail. It didn't take long for the savings to deplete entirely. We were fortunate to have Jenna's parents generously helping us with some of the payments, but we were adults who were bringing in very good salaries. Call it pride or a need to be self-sufficient, but I didn't want to rely on my in-laws for money as if I were a teenager depending on an allowance."

—Mike

If you are fortunate, you may have parents or other family members who are both willing and able to give a gift toward your infertility treatment. As of 2007, you can give a gift of up to $12,000 per person and avoid a gift tax. If they do so, you may want to discuss what you both want in terms of offering information as your treatment progresses. For example, would you prefer not to be asked what's happening on a daily basis?

If you aren't comfortable asking for a gift, perhaps if you ask for a loan, they may surprise you. Make a list of friends and/or family members you could ask for a loan. If you do, you can definitely beat credit card rates and probably those of any other commercial lender. But you still need to make it official. Sit down together and make a written loan plan, including interest rate and payment schedule.

Credit Card Debt

"My husband and I have been undergoing infertility treatment for several years. Unfortunately, we don't have insurance coverage, so most has been out of pocket for us. We did several rounds of Clomid, several injectable/IUI, three fresh IVFs, and one FET. Unfortunately, all we have to show for it is two miscarriages and a lot of debt. We used health savings accounts, credit cards, and a home equity line to fund all of our treatments. We have just moved on to adoption and are using our home equity line to finance that."

—Sydney

Credit card debt is one the most dangerous hazards in infertility debt. Credit cards are fairly easy to get and easy to use. It is not uncommon to max out your credit cards during infertility treatments. Since interest rates can range from 7 percent to 23 percent, with no tax benefits, this needs to be the last resort. Credit card borrowers must read the entire terms and conditions, and be aware of attractive teasers and future changes in terms with damaging long-term consequences if the conditions are not met precisely.

If you need to use credit cards, choose the right one. For example, some cards will give you 5 percent back on pharmacy, gas, and supermarket purchases. You'll be spending $2,000 on the meds alone—so that's $100 back. There are literally hundreds of different types of credit cards, offering everything from cash rebates to hotel rewards, airline miles and gasoline. Browse online and look for websites that offer extensive summaries of different credit card offers. Research the details carefully and apply online.

Top Ten List of Features to Consider When Selecting a Credit Card
1. Introductory APRs
2. Regular APR
3. Annual fees
4. Closure or early payoff fees
5. Overseas transactions fees
6. Late payment fees
7. Fees for cash advances

8. Types of interest (fixed or variable)
9. Credit limit
10. Types of rebates or cash-back programs

You do not have to shun credit cards completely, but you must keep track of them. Check on your credit card balances often. Always be aware of how much money you have charged and compare that with how much money you have in the bank. Don't use the credit card as though it were cash. Avoid charging more money than you have available. To avoid interest and service charges, don't carry a balance. Obviously not everyone can do this, but know that outstanding debt tends to cause more debt.

Home-Equity Debt

Home refinancing, home-equity loans, or lines of credit (also known as HELOC) are other types of personal loans that you can obtain to assist in paying for IVF treatment. Home-equity loans and HELOCs are slightly different. While they both use your home as collateral, home-equity loans give you a lump-sum payment (usually electronically deposited into a checking account), while a HELOC allows you to receive convenience checks as needed. Many lenders set the credit limit on a HELOC by taking a certain percentage of the home's appraised value and subtracting from the balanced owed on the existing mortgage.

What to Look for When Comparing HELOC Offers

Don't assume your mortgage company is going to offer you the best deal. When comparing HELOC offers, you need to compare apples to apples.

1. Introductory rate and period
2. Margin
3. Minimum draw
4. Required average balance
5. Up-front lender fees
6. Up-front third-party fees
7. Annual fee
8. Cancelation fee

In general, utilizing a home equity loan is preferable to other forms of debt. The interest rates tend to be lower than with other loans, and there is a lower up-front cash outlay in terms of fees, closing costs, and interest rates. Also, this type of equity line of credit would provide a potential tax deduction for interest paid on the borrowed amount. The major risk is that you're putting your home on the line if you can't make the payments. Think carefully about this one before you sign on the dotted line.

Retirement Savings

Many of us have 401(k) or other retirement savings plans through our work. A 401(k) plan allows a worker to save for retirement while deferring income taxes on the saved money and earnings until withdrawal. The employee elects to have a portion of his or her wage paid directly, or deferred, into his or her 401(k) account. For most of us, retirement seems so far away and that cash looks mighty attractive when we are trying to come up with money for infertility treatments. You are not alone. Studies have shown that nearly half of workers cash out of their 401(k) plans at some point.

Virtually all employers impose severe restrictions on withdrawals while a person continues to work at the company and is under age fifty-nine and a half. Any withdrawal that is permitted before age fifty-nine and a half is subject to an excise tax equal to 10 percent of the amount distributed in addition to any income taxes owed. This includes withdrawals made to pay for expenses due to a hardship. The tax code defines a hardship as medical expenses not covered by insurance for the employee, their spouse, or dependent(s), and this can include infertility.

Plans also allow employees to take loans from their 401(k) to be repaid with after-tax funds at predefined interest rates. The interest proceeds then become part of the 401(k) balance. The loan itself is not taxable income nor subject to the 10 percent penalty as long as it is paid back in accordance with section 72(p) of the Internal Revenue Code. This section requires, among other things, that the loan be for a term no longer than five years (except for the purchase of a primary residence), that a "reasonable" rate of interest be charged, and that substantially equal payments (with payments made at least every calendar quarter) be made over the life of the loan.

Employers, of course, have the option to make their plan's loan provisions more restrictive. When an employee does not make payments in accordance with the plan or IRS regulations, the outstanding loan balance will be declared in "default." A defaulted loan, and possibly accrued interest on the loan balance, becomes a taxable distribution to the employee in the year of default with all the same tax penalties and implications of a withdrawal.

Cashing out your retirement savings completely should generally be considered a last resort. If you withdraw all your funds, you'll end up eroding one of your principal sources of retirement income. This is hard to make up. You can't delay the inevitable, and one day you will be in a situation where you will need this retirement savings.

Flexible Spending Accounts

A flexible spending account (FSA) is a tax-advantaged financial account that can be set up through your employer. An FSA allows you to set aside a portion of your earnings to pay for a qualified expense, such as for qualified medical expenses. All items must be intended to treat or prevent a specific medical condition, including facilitating a pregnancy and overcoming infertility. For more info on FSAs, read the IRS Publication 502 at http:// www.irs.gov/publications/p502/index.html.

The money deducted from your pay to put into a FSA is not subject to payroll taxes, resulting in a substantial tax savings. For example, if a person is in the 28 percent federal marginal tax bracket and must pay a 4 percent state tax (along with FICA taxes of typically 7.65 percent), taxes eat up about 40 percent of one's paycheck. If you deduct $2,000 and put that money into an FSA, this could save you almost $800 in tax savings. And some states even offer statewide deductions for contributions to these accounts.

The annual cap for a medical FSA varies by employer. Although the IRS cap is $5,000, the employer can set its own cap at much lower amounts. This minimizes their perceived risk for prefunding should the employee leave or be terminated. If the employee can no longer pay into the plan, the employer does not recapture their prefunding amount from the employee's payroll deduction.

One major drawback is that all money put into the FSA must be spent within the "plan year" as defined by your employer. Any money that is left unspent at the end of the year is forfeited back to the company. This is commonly referred to as the "use it or lose it" rule. All applications for refunds must be made by the date defined by your company as well.

In recent years, some companies have implemented a FSA debit card to allow employees access to their FSA directly. This also simplifies the labor-intensive claims processing and enhances the effect of prefunding medical FSAs. If your company does not offer a debit card, you are responsible to collect all receipts and bills and submit them to your employer.

FSA-Friendly Companies

- You can find a list of expenses allowed by most FSA plans at www.wageworks.com.
- CVS customers who use the CVS ExtraCare customer loyalty card can track purchases of FSA eligible products at www.cvs.com/flex.
- Drugstore.com places icons next to items on its website that are typically eligible for reimbursement under FSA guidelines.

Health Savings Accounts

Health savings accounts (HSAs) are slightly different than FSAs. An HSA is a tax-sheltered savings account similar to the IRA but earmarked for medical expenses. Deposits are 100 percent tax-deductible and can be withdrawn by check or debit card to pay routine medical bills with tax-free dollars. HSAs are helpful only if you have a low-cost, high-deductible health insurance policy. When combined with this type of health insurance plan, the HSA is meant to replace a traditional high-cost health insurance policy (with its low copays and mountains of restrictions on medical choices). What is not used from the account each year stays in the account and continues to grow interest on a tax-favored basis to supplement retirement, just like an IRA. Think of it as a medical IRA.

Deferred Compensation Plans

If you are employed by a tax-exempt employer, such as a state or local government, you might be able to take advantage of a deferred compensation plan as outlined in Section 457 of the IRS Code. Some of these plans allow employees to defer income tax on retirement savings. If you are eligible, you can defer up to $15,000 and then an additional $500 each year to account for cost-of-living adjustments. While most plans do not allow you to withdraw money early from this savings, you may be able to do so in the event of an "unforeseeable emergency" such as infertility or family building. This money could then be used toward infertility treatments.

Check with your benefits representative to determine if this option is appropriate for you. As frustrating as it is, don't be surprised if they don't understand what you are talking about or deny your request at first. Departments and agencies still view infertility as an "elective medical treatment." If you are denied, don't be discouraged. You will need to clearly point out that infertility does fall squarely within the definition of an "unforeseeable emergency" set forth by the IRS regulations. For instance, you should maintain that infertility does constitute a "sudden and unexpected illness." Also, you will need to establish that obtaining infertility treatments would present a financial hardship for you and your family. With a little hard work, you should be able to convince your employer that you do qualify for this type of deferred compensation plan. After all, the law is on your side.

Medical Tax Deduction Benefits

Most people incur medical expenses throughout the year, but they do not realize they can receive a tax deduction from them. This can result in saving huge amounts of money. As long as the total medical costs are more than 7.5 percent of your gross income, you can qualify for a tax deduction. This is easy to do since it is not uncommon for infertility-related expenses to exceed $20,000 in out-of-pocket costs in a single year. For $20,000 to be 7.5 percent of your gross income, you just need to make less than $270,000. Most of us certainly fall within this range.

Of course, as with all tax deductions, a few other rules apply. To fully take advantage of this deduction, document every medical expense paid out of pocket on your tax return for all members of your family. Don't forget to add up your dental and optometry bills as well as medication costs. You might even be able to deduct those stupid home pregnancy tests if you work with a knowledgeable accountant.

The cost of transportation can even be considered part of the tax deduction entitlement. If you calculate your cents-per-mile according to the IRS website, you can save even more money. All infertility treatments and infertility treatment–related expenses are entirely appropriate for these deductions. Exceptions include things like cosmetic surgery, bottled water, gym membership, teeth whitening, maternity clothes, and diaper services.

Keep careful records of your bills and receipts so you can take the biggest advantage from this tax deduction. With the outrageous cost of infertility treatments, who wouldn't benefit from the tax benefits that are available?

Determining Your Limits

> *"This experience has made us increasingly aware of how important it was to follow a budget and prioritize our goals in life. We are willing to sacrifice a lot, but we can't sacrifice any hope of a future—or even a home—if this doesn't work out for us the way we want it to. We are finally willing to accept there is more than one way to bring a child into our lives."*
>
> —Tim

Popular financial experts ranging from Suze Orman to Clark Howard differ drastically in their views about how to finance infertility. Some conclude that you should never, ever go into debt to have a child, while others say you can't put a price tag on your family. It's a tough call. Only you know what's best for you and your family. We believe that everyone has the right to have a child, but we certainly don't want you to end up having to pay for the rest of your life. Be smart and consider both the short-term and the long-term impact on your financial future.

Five Things You Can Do Right Now

1. Review your clinic's financing options, including multiple-treatment plan programs and payment plans.
2. Start a medical deduction tax file immediately. Review your employers' FSA options and increase your participation to the maximum level.

3. Consider changing credit cards if you're going to have to break one out.

4. Get a free copy of your credit report and confirm all the information. Incorrect data could cost you hundreds of dollars in higher interest fees for loans or credit cards.

5. Make a list of your monthly expenses, divided into fixed payments that you must make (car and house payments, telephone, food, electricity, et cetera) and variable payments (what you do not have to spend: entertainment, going out to eat, et cetera). See if there are ways to cut down on your variable payments now to increase savings and free cash flow.

CHAPTER 13

Beyond Treatment:
Explore Adoption

"A drive in our hearts is what brought us to step beyond treatments. We had always had a love for children, and since we can't afford to keep going with treatments, we stepped into the reality of adoption. The longing in my heart to share my love of life and education leads me to our journey into adoption. That is how we knew what to do next after that last miscarriage. I know it is hard to know what the line is and when that is, but all I can say is you will know. Money? Time? Love? All of it played a factor in our decision."

—TINA

WHILE ADOPTION IS NOT A cure for infertility, it is a wonderful option for many people interested in building their families. Between 30,000 and 40,000 infants and very young children are placed for adoption in the United States every year. Another 21,000 families annually adopt internationally. The Evan B. Donaldson Adoption Institute estimates between 2 percent and 4 percent of all families have adopted. While it takes time and isn't free, adoption may be a part of how you decide to build your family.

If infertility treatments don't work, you will want to have funds to pursue other avenues for becoming a parent. Once you decide how much money you have available to spend, you may decide to allocate a portion of your available resources toward adoption. With a lot of planning and research about the different types of adoptions and available resources, you can develop a realistic budget and a timeline.

What Does It Really Cost to Adopt?

Adding a child to your family by adoption can vary in cost from very little to more than $40,000. Most adoptions involve spending between $10,000

ADOPTION COST FACTORS

- Type of adoption

- Where the adoption occurs

- Country of origin of a foreign-born child

- Whether or not the agency charges a sliding-scale fee based on family income

- Amount of state or federal subsidy available for a child with special needs

- Federal or state tax credits available for reimbursement of adoption expenses

- Employer adoption benefits

- State reimbursement for nonrecurring expenses for the adoption of a child with special needs

---

and $20,000. There are a variety of ways to adopt a child, each of which comes with a different price tag. Let's look at some of the different ways to adopt a child.

RANGE OF ADOPTION COSTS

Foster Care Adoptions: $0 to $2,500
Independent Adoptions (Domestic): $8,000 to $25,000+
Licensed Private Agency Adoptions (Domestic): $5,000 to $40,000+
International Adoptions: $7,000 to $40,000+

Domestic Adoptions

"I don't think most people even know that the vast majority of domestic adoptions go through without a hitch. I have adopted four times with very little trouble; yet I have people telling me all of the time that domestic adoptions just don't happen anymore. What we

spent on the four adoptions was what it would have cost for us to adopt one child from Cambodia or Korea."

—LAURA

When you adopt in the United States, you have three basic options: using a state or public agency, using a private agency, or arranging the adoption yourself.

FOSTER CARE OR PUBLIC AGENCY ADOPTIONS

Adopting from the US foster care system is generally the least expensive type of adoption, usually involving little or no cost, and states provide subsidies to parents who adopt in this manner. These are commonly referred to as foster-to-adopt programs. More than one million children are in the foster care system, and according to adoption expert Carolyn Berger, social worker and adoption coordinator, estimates vary widely, but range from 114,000 to 500,000 children in foster care available for adoption. They are of all races, ethnicities, and ages. There may be a long wait for a newborn, but it is possible. Most foster care children are older or have special needs.

When adopting through a public agency, your fees will be very low because these adoptions are supported by state and federal tax dollars. The home study–parent preparation process involves a significant investment of time, but little investment of money. In some states even the legal costs of finalizing a public agency adoption are covered by the state. Other states charge a small fee for a home study, primarily to establish a commitment on the part of the person asking to adopt. In some states, families are required to hire their own attorney to finalize a public agency adoption. For most of these cases, the legal paperwork involved is so routine, the costs of such a finalization usually involves just a few billable hours.

INDEPENDENT ADOPTIONS

"It's heartbreaking to consider giving up your dream of a family because of money. But that's where we were. We chose to skip IVF and go directly to adoption, and it was a financial challenge the whole way. A close friend of mine steered us in the direction of private adoption through an attorney—and it was the best decision

we ever made. If done with care and knowledge, it can be done
without costing too much. We had to do more work on our own, but
we didn't have to come up with the $10,000 that the private
agency wanted just to get us on the list."

—ELAINE

An independent adoption is a legal method of building a family without using an adoption agency for placement. In an independent adoption, the birth parents relinquish their parental rights directly to the adoptive parents instead of to an agency. And the prospective parents, in conjunction with an experienced adoption attorney, take an active role in identifying a birth mother, usually by networking, advertising, or using the internet.

Independent adoptions are attractive to birth parents and prospective adoptive parents because they allow the people involved to keep control over the adoption process. Adoptive parents are reassured by knowing the birth parents personally and dealing with them directly, instead of being afraid that their adoption may fall apart before it is completed. Rather than relying on an agency as a go-between, the birth parent and adoptive parents can meet, get to know each other, and decide for themselves whether to go ahead with the adoption. Independent adoptions also avoid the long waiting lists and restrictive qualifying criteria that can be part of agency adoptions. And independent adoptions usually happen much faster than agency adoptions, often within a year of beginning the search for a child. Finally, independent adoptions can be less expensive than using an agency; although the adoptive parents will have similar costs, like paying the birth mother's expenses, they will save the agency fees.

On the other hand, there are some downsides. States place significant restrictions on independent adoptions. For example, states may prohibit adoptive parents from advertising for a birth mother or limit the amount of money adoptive parents can contribute to the birth mother's prenatal care and medical expenses. Another concern is that birth parents might not receive adequate counseling during the adoption process. States differ quite a bit on how much counseling they require birth parents to have before making their final decision to place a child for adoption. If the birth parents do not get the required amount of counseling, this may make your adoption agreement vulnerable.

Adoptive families who pursue independent adoptions report spending $8,000 to $25,000 or more, depending on several factors. Independent adoptions are now allowed in most states, but advertising in newspapers, magazines, or the internet seeking birth parents is not allowed in all states. Costs for advertising for birth parents can be in the $5,000 range. Unlike agency fees, which are generally fixed and known in advance, the costs of independent adoption vary and depend on several factors. These include legal fees; a home study by a licensed professional; advertising expenses; travel costs (if applicable); and possibly counseling and/or medical expenses for the birth mother and child—depending on the nature of her insurance coverage, if any.

"Because adoption is, for the most part, controlled by state law, you will want to engage an experienced adoption attorney," explains Mark T. McDermott, an adoption attorney and adoptive parent. "But do not, in any circumstances, pay an adoption facilitator, pay someone to do your advertising for you, or pay a coach to tell you how to do the basics. If you are willing to do the legwork, you can control your costs."

Sample Domestic Adoption Expenses

COST	LOW	HIGH
AGENCY FEES		
Application fee	$100	$500
Home study and preparation services	$700	$2,500
Postplacement supervision	$200	$1,500
Parent physical (each parent)	$35	$150
Psychiatric evaluation (each parent, if required)	$250	$400
ATTORNEY FEES		
Document preparation	$500	$2,000
Petition and court representation to finalize placement	$2,500	$12,000

COST	LOW	HIGH
ADVERTISING	$500	$5,000

BIRTH PARENT EXPENSES	Amount and type of expenses allowable for payment usually restricted by state law and subject to review by the court.	
Medical expenses (prenatal, birth and delivery, postnatal for mother; perinatal care for child)	$0 (insurance)	$10,000–$20,000 (depending on difficulty of the delivery, et cetera)
Living expenses (rent, food, clothing, transportation, et cetera)	$500	$12,000
Legal representation	$500	$1,500
Counseling	$500	$2,000

With an independent adoption, you may need to come up with money quickly. "We had an unexpected situation. We thought we had six to nine months to come up with the cash for the adoption, but within a month we were called about a baby boy," explains Terri, an adoptive mom. "We used a zero-percent credit card and paid it off prior to the due date. It was like a loan that was interest free. We also borrowed against our retirement fund with no penalties or fees. The repayment is low, and we repay out of each check so we don't notice it. Creative financing can go a long way."

You have to work at any type of adoption you pursue, so if you aren't afraid of rolling up your sleeves and getting invested in the process, this is the way to go. Adoption forums and support groups are good places to start collecting information, and they can refer you to the best, most current resources.

LICENSED PRIVATE AGENCY ADOPTIONS

An agency adoption is arranged through a child placement agency. Agencies are experienced in finding children, matching them with parents, and satisfying the necessary legal requirements. The most important factor in selecting an agency is that they have met the requirements of your state and are fully licensed to provide you with a full range of professional services. To check if an agency or organization is licensed, contact them and ask for their license number and the phone number of the licensing authority. Then call the authority and confirm that the information given to you is correct.

In private agency adoptions, birth parents relinquish their parental rights to the agency before the baby is placed with the adoptive parents. Adoptions can be closed or open. In a closed child adoption, the birth parents and adopting family are anonymous. While details may be shared, no identifying information (such as last name, addresses, Social Security numbers, et cetera) is exchanged. The birth parents and adopting family can meet, share pictures and updates, and have ongoing contact through the agency, but they do not share last names and addresses. In an open child adoption, the biological and adopting parents exchange identifying information and are then able, if they so choose, to be in contact with one another directly. The key advantage of a private agency adoption is the extensive counseling that agencies provide. Typically, counseling is available for adoptive parents, birth parents, and the children (if they are older).

With a private agency, an adoptive family works directly with the agency and not the birth parents. Private agency social workers facilitate the match of a child and prospective adoptive parent. Agencies may give preference to certain types of individuals or couples based on faith, age, income level, health, family size, marital status, or personal history (including criminal records). The wait for an infant through a licensed private agency varies from several months to a few years. Expenses for agency adoptions can easily reach $40,000, but they are generally predictable and are outlined up front by the adoption agency. "Private agency adoptions cost more, you have less control over the process, it takes longer, and agreements are sometimes broken by birth moms with agencies because they aren't dealing with you as adoptive parents; they are dealing with a bureaucracy," explains McDermott.

International Adoption

When children are adopted from outside the United States, it is known as international adoption. There are approximately fifty countries throughout the world from which children can be adopted. Although you can get help through an adoption agency specializing in international adoptions, this type of adoption is essentially a legal matter between a private individual (or couple) who wishes to adopt and a foreign court, which operates under that country's laws and regulations. International adoption costs vary greatly according to the specific laws of the foreign country from which you are adopting. Let's look more closely at some of the specifics:

Costs can vary according to many factors, including:

- Whether the foreign country is a participant in the Hague Convention, which ensures the protection of children with regard to intercountry adoption (for more information about the Hague Convention, visit the US Department of State at www.travel.state.gov).
- Whether the placement entities in the foreign country are government agencies, government-subsidized orphanages, charitable foundations, attorneys, facilitators, or any combination of these.
- Whether the foreign country requires translation and/or authentication of the dossier documents.
- Whether the US agency requires a "donation" to the foreign orphanage or agency.
- Whether the foreign agency requires one or both adoptive parents to travel to the country for interviews and court hearings; this could be one or more trips of varying length.

STATE DEPARTMENT FEES

Your own government doesn't make it any cheaper to adopt internationally. Not included in your adoption agency fees are the charges by the US government for processing all the federal forms and visa applications—the total cost for processing all these forms is around $1,000. This does not include incidental charges for passports, local requirements such as state or county fingerprinting, and mailing costs.

The Office of Children's Issues in the Bureau of Consular Affairs provides brochures describing the adoption process in numerous countries. In addition, they provide recorded information on intercountry adoption for several countries on a twenty-four-hour basis through their recorded telephone messages at 1-888-407-4747.

Agency Fees

Expect to pay somewhere between $7,000 and $40,000. The agency fees really do vary this much. Some adoption agencies may lower their fees for families adopting older children or children with special needs and for lower-income families. Also, families with a member in full-time ministry may receive a discount when applying with a religious-based agency. They will also typically lower their fees for adopting multiple children at a time or for repeat clients. Even if the agency doesn't offer to lower its fee, you should always ask.

Agency fees include:

- INS/State Department visa application, processing, and visa medical fees
- Home study and parent preparation
- Psychological evaluations (if required)
- Physical examinations
- Postplacement supervision (if required)
- Translation and authentication of adoption dossier documents (if required)
- Agency placement fee

Fees in the Foreign Country

Travel expenses can add up quickly. Because arrangements can change quickly, assume you aren't going to get a super bargain on your airfare. Adoption.com explains, "To get a decent estimate once you've chosen a country, see what ticket prices are for two weeks' advance notice for travel to get there. Also check for special adoption fares from the airlines. (And remember that some countries require you to travel twice!) And if you're adopting a toddler or older child, you also need to remember to add in the cost of a one-way ticket for your new child for the way back. Aside from airfare, the hotel bills and meals can really add up quickly, so add this into your cost estimate."

Travel expenses can include:

- Transportation, hotel, meals
- Foreign agency placement fee

- Foreign attorney legal and placement fee
- Foster and medical care for the child
- Use of translation and escort services by US agency representative in the foreign country
- Foreign court filing fee and document fees (birth certificate and adoption decree)
- Required "donation" to orphanage or agency
- Translation services and escort services
- Passport office fees

Home Study

If you live in the United States and plan to adopt, you will need an adoption home study. States require home studies before a child can be placed in your custody. It is recommended that you complete a home study as one of the first steps in your adoption process. Home study requirements vary, but generally an adoption caseworker will have you submit an intake form and interview you to help her evaluate if you are qualified to adopt according to the guidelines of your state. Usually background checks, financial reviews, and at least one home visit are part of the process.

The home study will typically cost anywhere from $300 to $3,000 (not including postplacement visits, which can cost around $200 per visit). International home study preparers are licensed differently than social workers who perform domestic adoption home studies, so work with an experienced agency.

Your Finances

"I was worried that we would be rejected because of a bankruptcy years ago, but we weren't required to have an actual credit report done. We just had to list all of our major regular payments: house, cars, student loans, et cetera. And then you give them an income statement. For us it was a copy of our W2s from the previous year. Basically they were interested in our debt-to-income ratio. Did we have enough money to support one more member of the family?"

—MARY BETH

"You will be sharing rather intimate financial information as part of a home study," explains Patricia Irwin Johnston, an adoptive mother and author of *Adoption: Sound Choices, Strong Families*. "A credit check will be run; your employment will be verified; tax records for recent years may be requested. Agencies are not looking for wealth, but for reasonable and responsible financial management. Low debt ratio speaks more highly of those who want to be parents than do assets secured by large mortgages, loans, and credit card debt."

Parenting is an expensive proposition, no matter who you are. Agencies and birth parents want to be reassured you understand this and have planned for it. They will ask questions about the number of hours you work and about your plans for day care. They will ask you to explore your health insurance benefits and may require that one parent be able to stay home for at least half a year. "The bottom line is that anyone planning to become a parent through adoption will need to have taken a careful look at their budget and adjusted it and their life accordingly," says Johnston.

Financial Help

While adoption can be an expensive endeavor, you have some options to help defray your expenses.

DEPENDENCY EXEMPTIONS

Adoptive parents are eligible for federal and state dependency tax exemption for their adopted children. The amount of exemption is adjusted annually and helps by reducing your taxable income.

If your child is placed with you, but the adoption is not finalized until the following year, you can still claim a tax deduction for the child *as your dependent* in the year he or she was placed with you—even though the adoption was not finalized at that time. Children whose adoptions have been finalized are eligible for the same exemptions as a biological child.

FEDERAL TAX CREDIT

The federal adoption tax credit is more beneficial than a simple tax deduction. Under the Hope for Children Act (Public Law 107–16) "qualifying adoption expenses" up to $11,390 (for families with gross incomes under

$170,8205) may be deducted from overall federal tax liability. Qualified adoption expenses must be legal and may include adoption fees, attorney fees, birth parent expenses and travel costs, including necessary transportation, meals, and lodging.

Be sure you fully understand the difference between a tax deduction and a tax credit. If you are not paying $11,390 per year in taxes, you will not get a full $11,390 credit in one year. However, you can spread out the tax credit over five years, if necessary. In addition, you can take two years to take full advantage of the tax credit. For example, if your federal tax obligation is $6,000 and you have $4,000 in adoption expenses, your tax liability would be reduced to $2,000. If your tax bill is smaller than the amount of your expenses, you can carry forward the unused portion of your adoption tax credit for the next several years.

If your domestic adoption falls through, you can still apply for the tax credit. However, you can claim only one credit per "attempt." You cannot claim for a failed international adoption.

STATE BENEFITS

Some states offer a tax credit or deduction in addition to the federal tax credit. Such states offer a deduction up to $5,000. Check your state's tax laws for details on tax deductions or tax credits for adoptions. And remember, tax deductions are not as big a savings as tax credits.

States That Offer Tax Assistance for Adoption

- Arizona
- California
- Idaho
- Iowa
- Kansas
- Maryland
- Massachusetts
- Michigan
- Missouri
- New Mexico
- North Dakota
- Oklahoma

- Utah
- West Virginia
- Wisconsin

Employee Benefits

At least 25 percent of corporations in the United States offer some form of adoption benefits to their employees. Typical benefits may include reimbursement of adoption expenses (typically $1,000 to $10,000); paid leave in addition to vacation time, sick leave, or personal days; and unpaid leave.

Even if your employer doesn't currently offer adoption benefits, ask about their availability. You may be able to persuade your company to begin offering them. Work with other employees interested in adoption, gather information for the employer, and present your case. Also, find out if your employer offers an Employee Assistance Program (EAP). This benefit was designed to help employees deal with dramatic personal situations or problems. For more information about employer benefits, including materials to help you request that your employer establish a program, call the National Adoption Center at 1-800-TO-ADOPT.

Subsidies

Families who adopt children domestically with special medical, emotional, and/or developmental needs, older children, or members of a sibling group may find that their children are eligible for an adoption subsidy from federal and state governments. Subsidies are used to cover special education, health, and therapeutic needs of children with special needs. You may be able to negotiate a conditional subsidy in case problems arise later on.

Unless an international adoption goes awry, throwing the child into the US child welfare system, internationally adopted children are not typically eligible for these subsidies. Check with your state government or social worker for details, and don't accept a first "no" answer. Subsidies are for the benefit of children, and they are not based on family financial need, but on the needs of the child, so it is important to be a strong advocate for yourself and your child.

MILITARY SUBSIDIES

After an adoption has been finalized, active-duty military personnel can receive reimbursement per child up to $2,000 for adoption-related expenses, up to a maximum of $5,000 in one year. Reimbursement does not include travel costs, but it does include medical costs for a birth mother and the child.

FRIENDS AND FAMILY

"Another way that you can help us is by donating your loose change. Anyone interested in this method will be provided with a decorated baby bottle to place the spare change in. When it is full, or you would like to bless us, you can send it back to us. We also have a stuffed animal we have available for a $10.00 donation. His shirt says, 'I Support Adoption.'"

—TIFFANY in her web page appeal for financial support

The same strategies mentioned in earlier chapters can still be effective if you pursue adoption. In fact, as we mentioned earlier, raising money for adoption expenses may be significantly easier than doing so for infertility treatment.

How to Save Money When Adopting

- Read your adoption agreement and contracts carefully.
- Make decisions from your head and heart together.
- Complete necessary paperwork in a timely manner.
- Don't use an adoption facilitator (instead use a licensed adoption agency).
- Do extensive research on any adoption professionals and agencies you decide to work with.

CONCLUSIONS

"We recently adopted and we have our hands full with an active toddler. I'm finally happy, content, and a parent. I'm glad I did so many cycles, 'cause at least now I know that my chances are so grim that another cycle isn't going to give me the result I want. Donor egg didn't really appeal to me, and now that I have my darling daughter, I feel like our family is complete."

—PAULA

The emotional process of moving toward adoption can be very difficult. Dr. Janet Jaffe, director of the Center for Reproductive Psychology and coauthor of *Unsung Lullabies: Understanding and Coping with Infertility*, explains: "If you see a dress in a window, you don't know how it looks until you try it on. Try to do the same thing psychologically. Imagine what life would look like with your partner if you didn't have children five years from now. Imagine what life would feel like if you adopted internationally. Think about it. What would life be like if you decide to invest in the lives of children in other ways? Try it on to see how it fits. There are no right or wrong answers; each individual and each couple must come to their own conclusion.

"Sometimes people will jump into adoption before they are ready to do that because they can't afford another IVF cycle. And the truth is, they are not emotionally and psychologically ready. It becomes a secondary or somewhat lesser choice. Any decision you make about building your family needs to be a first choice. And it may take some time to get there."

> *"I am grateful for my infertility. I'm grateful that it kept us from making a baby and missing out on my daughter Madison. I'm grateful my life led me to adoption, to Jessica [Madison's birth mom], and to a new understanding of motherhood. I am humbled by the privilege of being part of the triad, and I know that the whole experience made me a better woman. I know it must sound strange, but I feel pretty lucky to have been infertile."*
>
> —MONA

Five Things You Can Do Right Now

1. If adoption interests you, check out your state's laws at www.theadoptionguide.com.
2. Review your and your partner's benefits package to determine if adoption benefits are included in your compensation.
3. Seek out the most recent comprehensive resources on adoption.
4. Start a list of possible agencies and attorneys you may be interested in.
5. Check out others' experiences with specific adoption professionals at fertilethoughts.com.

CHAPTER 14

Breaking Down Barriers:
Final Thoughts

"As we snuggled into bed last night, my husband, insane but wonderful man that he is, suddenly announced: 'Choo-choo . . . All aboard the crazy train!' Ah—finally he understood the misery that was coming next in the form of the two-week wait. It's the last IVF we can afford. He knows how hard the next few weeks will be.

"And it is hard to imagine anything good coming from the hell we call infertility. But it has. This journey has shown me what a fantastic husband I have. He doesn't flinch when I'm in the stirrups and the man in white comes at me with a new torture device. He tells me we will be parents, he assures me we'll find the money for what we need, and he protects me from my mother-in-law's nosy questions. I am grateful for him. I never needed him before the way I do now. At least when we get to other side of this journey, whatever that looks like, I won't be alone."

—NORA

"MOST OF US BELIEVE WE'LL get pregnant and have a baby without a hitch. That's the way it's supposed to be," says Dr. Janet Jaffe. "But when these hopes and dreams crumble, you may feel as if your whole world is falling apart. You may feel confused, get angry, and grieve. You enter the ups and downs of medical treatment, turning the control of your reproductive life over to the custody of your doctors. What's so important to remember in this crazy journey you have entered is that no matter what, you are more than your reproductive self. Sometimes, in your helplessness, you may forget that you are a strong and vital person, productive in so many other areas of life."

Your desire to create a family has gone in directions you never imagined, you still have the power to decide the course it will take. You may not know exactly how you'll get to your final destination—whether IVF will finally work, whether adoption is the answer, whether you will use donor technology, or whether you will continue as a family of two—but you are in the driver's seat and you will get through this.

Moving through infertility with unexpected delays and detours is just one part of your whole life. You can make choices to minimize the damage from the potholes, landslides, and upheavals along the way, whether or not you have children. You have control over the steering wheel and the route you take so that will have the power to right the wrongs to your sense of self, your relationships, your plans, and your life.

The truth is out: We can't really wave our magic ultrasound wands and

TOP 10 MISTAKES WHEN IT COMES TO BUDGETING FOR INFERTILITY

1. Do what your fertility specialist tells you to do without question.
2. Accept what the doctor's office tells you about your insurance coverage.
3. Choose a fertility clinic because it's the one closest to your job.
4. Get your script filled at your local pharmacy (without comparing prices).
5. Keep sloppy billing and insurance records.
6. Continue on a treatment path that isn't working. A year of Clomid, anyone?
7. Refuse to consider other alternatives such as travel or clinical trials.
8. Accept your insurance company's claim denial without argument.
9. Ignore the HR department at your job as a potential advocate.
10. Begin treatment without a long-term plan and defined boundaries of time, energy, and/or money.

make all your financial woes disappear. Infertility treatment is expensive. And not just in terms of your pocketbook. It affects your family, job, relationships, and mental health. You'll need to weigh all of those factors when making decisions.

Now you are armed with the information and power you need to take control of your fertility plan. You can choose cost-effective treatment, create the best treatment team for you, save money on medications, and fight your insurance company for the coverage you deserve.

There isn't one right way to grow your family. Ultimately, the decisions you make will be the right ones for you. Be wise. Surround yourself with people who love, support, and encourage you. Get professional help when you need it. Be open and honest with your health care providers. Believe in your partner and be patient when you are at different places. Trust your "gut instincts." Above all, take care of yourself.

Helpful Websites and Organizations

ADOPTION

Adoption.com
➤ www.adoption.com

American Academy of Adoption Attorneys
➤ www.adoptionattorneys.org

Dave Thomas Foundation for Adoption
➤ www.davethomasfoundation.org

Evan B. Donaldson Adoption Institute
➤ www.adoptioninstitute.org

National Council for Adoption
➤ www.adoptioncouncil.org

Finding Your Child
➤ www.creatingafamily.com

North American Council on Adoptable Children
➤ www.nacac.org

Perspectives Press
➤ www.perspectivespress.com

ADOPTION GRANTS

Adoption Financing Information
➤ www.financinginformation.com

Affording Adoption
➤ www.affordingadoption.com

ART STATISTICS

Centers for Disease Control and Prevention
➤ www.cdc.gov/art

Society for Assisted Reproductive Technologies
➤ www.sart.org

BLOGS: ADOPTION

A Dad's Journey Through International Adoption
➤ http://frwl-fromdad.blogspot.com/

Adoption Blogs
➤ www.adoptionblogs.com

Belly Laughs and Crocodile Tears
➤ http://www.daisyface.blogspot.com/

Closed Door, Open Window (Foster Care to Adoption)
➤ http://closeddooropenwindow.blogspot.com/

Life with Ivan (International Adoption)
➤ http://a-leapof-faith.blogspot.com/

My Best Laid Plans
➤ http://www.mybestlaidplans.blogspot
.com/

They Grow in Your Heart
➤ http://theygrowinyourheart.blogspot
.com/

BLOGS: INFERTILITY

A Little Pregnant
➤ www.alittlepregnant.com

Stirrup Queens and Sperm Palace Jesters
➤ http://stirrup-queens.blogspot.com

Sarah Solitaire (Family Building When
Single)
➤ http://sarah-solitaire.blogspot.com/

Two Moms Are Better Than One (Gay and
Lesbian Family Building)
➤ http://twomomsarebetterthanone
.wordpress.com/

To Infertility and Beyond
➤ http://toinfertilityandbeyond.blogspot
.com/

CANCER AND FERTILITY

Fertile Hope
➤ www.fertilehope.org

FAMILIES OF COLOR

Ferre Institute
➤ www.infertilityeducation.org/
familiesofcolor.html

FERTILITY AWARENESS

Taking Charge of Your Fertility
➤ www.tcoyf.com

GAY AND LESBIAN FAMILIES

Family Equality Council
➤ www.familyequality.org

GENERAL INFORMATION ABOUT INFERTILITY

American Society for Reproductive
Medicine (ASRM)
➤ www.asrm.org

The Boston Women's Health Book
Collective
➤ www.ourbodiesourselves.org

WebMD
➤ www.webmd.com

GRANTS AND FINANCIAL ASSISTANCE: ADOPTION

The Gift of Adoption Fund
➤ www.giftofadoption.org

The National Adoption Foundation
➤ www.nafadopt.org

The Orphan Foundation
➤ www.theorphanfoundation.org

GRANTS AND FINANCIAL ASSISTANCE: INFERTILITY TREATMENTS

Cleveland Clinic Partnership for Families
➤ www.clevelandclinic.org/obgyn/

Fertile Dreams Organization
➤ www.fertiledreams.org

International Council on Infertility
Information Dissemination
(From INCIID the Heart Program)
➤ www.inciid.org

Jude Andrew Adams Charitable Fund
➤ www.lotusblossomconsulting.com

Tinina Q. Cade Foundation
➤ www.cadefoundation.org

HEALTH CARE ADVOCACY

Center for Patient Advocacy
➤ www.patientadvocacy.org

Consumer Coalition for Quality Health Care
➤ www.consumers.org

Consumer Watchdog: Protecting Patients
➤ www.consumerwatchdog.org

Joint Commission
➤ www.jcrinc.com

INFERTILITY PATIENT SUPPORT

A T.I.M.E. A Torah Infertility Medium of Exchange
➤ www.atime.org

Fertility Plus: Information Written by Patients, for Patients
➤ www.fertilityplus.org

My Fertile Ground
➤ www.myfertileground.com

INTERNATIONAL MEDICAL TRAVEL

European Society of Human Reproduction & Embryology
➤ www.eshre.com

Joint Commission International
➤ www.jointcommissioninternational.org

Medical Nomad
➤ www.medicalnomad.com

Medical Tourism
➤ www.MedicalTourism.com

Patients Beyond Borders
➤ www.patientsbeyondborders.com

MIND-BODY APPROACH

The Domar Center
➤ www.domarcenter.com

PERSONAL FINANCE

Saving Money & Personal Finance Advice
➤ www.savingadvice.com

Self Growth
➤ www.selfgrowth.com

Smart Money Advocate
➤ www.smartmoneyadvocate.com

PHARMACEUTICAL COMPANIES

Ferring Pharmaceuticals
➤ www.ferringfertility.com

Organon
➤ www.fertilityjourney.com

Serono
➤ www.fertilitylifelines.com

SINGLE MOTHERS

Choosing Single Motherhood
➤ www.choosingsinglemotherhood.com

THIRD-PARTY REPRODUCTION

American Surrogacy Center (Surrogacy and Egg Donor Information)
➤ www.surrogacy.com

Sperm Bank Directory
➤ www.spermbankdirectory.com

The Donor Sibling Registry
➤ www.donorsiblingregistry.com

Appendix 1: Creating Your Fertility Budget

How Much Money Do You Have to Work With?

CATEGORY	AMOUNT PAID MONTHLY
INCOME	
Wages and Bonuses	
Interest Income	
Investment Income (Savings, Retirement, Stocks, etc.)	
Miscellaneous Income (Gifts, etc.)	
Income Subtotal	
INCOME TAXES WITHHELD	
Federal Income Tax	
State and Local Income Tax	
Social Security, Medicare Tax	
Income Taxes Subtotal	
SPENDABLE INCOME PER MONTH	
SPENDABLE INCOME PER YEAR	

How Much Money Are You Spending?

CATEGORY	AMOUNT PAID MONTHLY	NEW PLANNED AMOUNT	SAVINGS
HOME			
Mortgage or Rent			
Home Owners/Renters Insurance			
Property Taxes			
Home Repairs, Maintenance, HOA Dues			
Home Improvements			
UTILITIES			
Electricity			
Water and Sewer			
Natural Gas or Oil			
Telephone (Land Line, Cell)			
Trash Removal			
Cable			
FOOD			
Groceries			
Eating Out, Lunches, Snacks			
FAMILY OBLIGATIONS			
Child Support, Alimony			
Day Care, Babysitting			
HEALTH AND MEDICAL			
Insurance (Medical, Dental, Vision)			
Out-of-Pocket Medical Expenses			
Fitness (Yoga, Massage, Gym)			
TRANSPORTATION			
Car Payments			
Gasoline, Oil			
Auto Repairs, Maintenance, Fees			
Auto Insurance			
Other (Tolls, Bus, Subway, Taxi)			

CATEGORY	AMOUNT PAID MONTHLY	NEW PLANNED AMOUNT	SAVINGS
DEBT PAYMENTS			
Credit Cards			
Student Loans			
Other Loans			
ENTERTAINMENT, RECREATION			
Cable TV, Videos, Movies			
Computer Expense			
Hobbies			
Subscriptions and Dues			
Vacations			
PETS			
Food			
Grooming, Boarding, Veterinarian			
CLOTHING			
INVESTMENTS AND SAVINGS			
401(k) or IRA			
Stocks, Bonds, Mutual Funds			
College Fund			
Savings			
Emergency Fund			
MISCELLANEOUS			
Toiletries, Household Products			
Gifts, Donations			
Grooming (Hair, Makeup, Other)			
Miscellaneous Expenses			
Total Investments and Expenses per Month			
Total Amount of Spendable Income per Month			
Total Amount of Surplus or Debt per Month			

Appendix 2: Creating Your Fertility Action Plan

This is your opportunity to begin keeping track of your goals and to prepare for decisions you may have to make while seeking treatment for infertility. These questions will help you focus on the medical, financial, and emotional aspects of trying to conceive.

CONSIDERING TREATMENT

- How long are you willing to try before moving to a fertility specialist?

- Do other health concerns need to be addressed before becoming pregnant?

- Because age plays an important role in fertility, how will your age affect your treatment decisions?

TREATMENT OPTIONS

- How do you feel about undergoing infertility treatments?

- Are there any kinds of treatments you aren't willing to undertake?

- How does undergoing fertility testing and treatments fit with your personal and religious beliefs?

- Between you and your partner, if applicable, discuss these options and consider how comfortable you might be with these if necessary:

  - Surgery
  - Medication only
  - IUI
  - IUI with medication

- In Vitro Fertilization
- ICSI
- Sperm Donor
- Egg Donor
- Embryo Donor
- PGD
- Surrogacy
- Egg/Embryo Freezing

- Do you and your partner agree about infertility treatments? What will you do if you do not agree?

TREATMENT LIMITS

- How many cycles are you willing to try for each treatment?

- How will you know that it is time to move on?

- If a treatment isn't completely successful, what other options would be?

  - Adoption
  - Foster care
  - Surrogacy
  - Child-free Living

FINANCIAL LIMITS

- What is and is not covered by your health insurance?

- How will you pay for tests and treatments not covered by insurance?

- How much can you spend out-of-pocket per month or per year?

- Do you have friends or family willing to loan or give you money? If so, how much?

- Are you willing to cash out retirement plans to fund infertility treatment?

Appendix 3: Evaluating Your Insurance Coverage

Knowing your coverage will help avoid misunderstandings. Review your plan documents and complete the following worksheet to (1) understand your coverage and (2) have the necessary information ready in a convenient place when you need to arrange care. What follows is a checklist to help you remember information about your coverage:

MY HEALTH PLAN COVERAGE IS THROUGH:

☐ My employer. Check if:

    ☐ my plan is an insured plan; any plan denials are eligible for state external review

    ☐ my plan is a self-funded plan; any plan denials are NOT eligible for state external review

☐ A policy I bought myself

☐ An association-sponsored policy (such as through a trade, civic, or educational organization)

☐ Other: _____

MY HEALTH PLAN IS A:

☐ Health maintenance organization (HMO)

☐ Preferred provider organization (PPO)

☐ Point-of-service plan (POS)

☐ Traditional indemnity (also known as fee-for-service)

Plan number to call if I have a problem: _____

My primary care physician is: _____

Physician's phone number: _____

I NEED A REFERRAL FROM MY PRIMARY CARE PHYSICIAN FOR:

☐ Lab and x-ray tests

☐ Gynecologist (for well-woman exam)

☐ Gynecologist (for other concerns)

☐ Pediatrician

☐ Other specialist visits

☐ Surgery

☐ Other: _____

MY PRIMARY CARE PHYSICIAN HAS THE FOLLOWING REQUIREMENTS FOR OBTAINING REFERRALS:

☐ Requires an office visit

☐ Requires _____ days' advance notice

☐ Other: _____

MY PRIMARY CARE PHYSICIAN CAN REFER ME TO SPECIALISTS WHO:

☐ Are part of his or her group practice

☐ Are on the health plan network list

☐ Are outside of the health plan network only if there are no similar specialists within the network

☐ Are outside of the health plan network

☐ I do not need a referral from my primary care physician

I HAVE REVIEWED THE EXCLUSIONS AND LIMITATIONS SECTION IN MY EVIDENCE OF COVERAGE. MY HEALTH PLAN WILL NOT PAY FOR, OR LIMITS, THE FOLLOWING SERVICES:

☐ _____

☐ _____

☐ _____

☐ _____

☐ _____

MY PLAN WILL COVER SERVICES AT THE FOLLOWING HOSPITALS:

_____

_____

_____

WHAT SHOULD I DO IF I NEED CARE WHILE I AM OUT OF MY PLAN'S SERVICE AREA?

For non-urgent care: _____

Phone: _____

In an urgent situation: _____

Phone: _____

In an emergency: _____

Phone: _____

IF YOU HAVE A PPO OR POS PLAN:

ALTHOUGH I CAN USE OUT-OF-NETWORK DOCTORS FOR MOST SERVICES, I *CANNOT* USE OUT-OF-NETWORK DOCTORS FOR THE FOLLOWING SERVICES:

☐ Mental health

☐ Substance abuse

☐ Other: _____

IF I USE OUT-OF-NETWORK PROVIDERS, I WILL PAY:

☐ $ _____ annual deductible

☐ _____ percent coinsurance for charges exceeding the deductible.

Appendix 4: Letter Requesting Predetermination of Benefits from Your Insurance Company

[Date]

[Your insurance company name and address]
RE: Predetermination of benefits for: [patient's name]
Group/Group Number: [name of group, if applicable]
ID Number: [patient's insurance identification number]

Dear [Insurance company contact name]:

My [husband, wife, partner] and I are considering [in vitro fertilization, gamete intrafallopian transfer, or other procedure your doctor has recommended]. This procedure is necessary to attempt pregnancy due to [explain your situation: e.g., blocked fallopian tubes, male factor, previous sterilization, unexplained infertility, etc.]. A fee schedule from our physician is attached for your review.

Please provide me with a written response to each of the questions below:

Is there a preexisting condition limitation?

Are separate referrals required for office visits, treatments cycles, medications, and surgical procedures?

Will [the procedure that applies to your situation] be a payable procedure under my current coverage or under my major medical portion?

If yes, is there a limit of any kind: dollars or number of attempts?

If no, are any portions of the charges payable [prescription medications, laboratory tests, ultrasounds, or any other components my doctor has identified]?

Is coverage dependent upon the use of certain pharmacies or laboratories?

To what extent does the plan cover support services, such as psychological counseling?

If none of the charges are payable, please identify the page in my contract where all charges are specifically excluded and the date the exclusion was added to the contract. If the charges are not excluded, I will assume they are payable.

I would appreciate a written response as soon as possible. Thank you. If you have any questions, please call [your phone number].

Sincerely,
[your name and address]

Appendix 5: Who to Contact Regarding a Health Plan Appeal

Who to call for an appeal: _____

Where to write for an appeal: _____

_____

_____

How soon must I appeal? _____

How many days will it take to receive a response? (List the response times for each level of review)

    1st level _____

    2nd level _____

    Expedited appeals (for medical emergencies) _____

_____

According to ERISA regulations, every employee benefit plan must establish and follow reasonable claims procedures. In order for the procedure to be deemed reasonable by the Department of Labor, it must include clear information about the entire appeal process, including all necessary documentation; the content of the benefit determination notifications and the manner by which it will be delivered to you; time frames; and how to deal with further appeals regarding any adverse benefits determinations. Ask your employer or human resource department for specific information about how to properly submit a health plan appeal before you start your fertility treatments.

Appendix 6: Letter Requesting Predetermination of Drug Coverage from Insurance Company

[Date]

[Your insurance company name/pharmacy benefit manager name and address]
RE: Predetermination of benefits for: [patient's name]
Group/Group Number: [name of group, if applicable]
ID Number: [patient's insurance identification number]

Dear [Insurance company contact name]:

My [husband, wife, partner] and I are considering infertility treatment. This procedure is necessary to attempt pregnancy due to [explain your situation: e.g., blocked fallopian tubes, male factor, previous sterilization, unexplained infertility, etc.]. Please provide me with a written response to each of the questions below:

Is there a preexisting condition limitation?

Are separate referrals required for office visits, treatments cycles, medications, and surgical procedures?

Which medications are covered by my medical plan?

_____ For ovulation induction (OI)?
_____ For intrauterine insemination (IUI)?
_____ For in vitro fertilization (IVF)?
_____ For gamete intrafallopian transfer (GIFT)?
_____ For zygote intrafallopian transfer (ZIFT)?
_____ For artificial insemination (AI)?
_____ For embryo transfer (ET)?

If covered under a pharmacy benefit, what is the copayment or deductible?

Is coverage dependent upon the use of certain pharmacies?

Is there a limit of any kind (dollars, time period, or number of cycles)?

If yes, are they lifetime limits or annual limits?

If none of the charges are payable, please identify the page in my contract where all charges are specifically excluded and the date the exclusion was added to the contract. If the charges are not excluded, I will assume they are payable.

I would appreciate a written response as soon as possible. Thank you. If you have any questions, please call [your phone number].

Sincerely,
[your name and address]

Appendix 7: Letter to Legislator for Insurance Coverage for Fertility Treatments

[Date]

[Your representative's name and address]
RE: [legislative bill number]

Dear Representative:

I am writing to express my support for [bill number], which is currently being considered. I urge you to support this bill, which seeks to establish insurance coverage for fertility treatment.

Currently, many insurance plans arbitrarily deny coverage for fertility, even though it is a recognized medical disease that can be effectively treated in most cases. [bill number] will remedy this unfair practice by offering coverage for fertility treatment. This coverage will provide appropriate treatment for infertile couples at a cost estimated to be less than [amount] per subscriber per year. [bill number] will give people like me the opportunity to build a family here in [your state] without putting an undue burden on others.

In states where there is no mandated coverage, individuals have been forced to turn to the court system to secure coverage for this medical condition.

The U.S. Equal Employment Opportunity Commission recently ruled in support of employer-provided infertility coverage. The EEOC ruled that a company violated the Americans with Disabilities Act and Title VII of the Civil Rights Act when it refused to pay for an employee's fertility treatment. In [your state], we think it is better to work through our legislature to provide an appropriate response to the inequities that exist under the current coverage scenarios.

I hope you will vote in favor of [bill number]. Thank you for your attention to this vital issue that affects me, my family members, friends, and coworkers.

Sincerely,
[your name, address, and phone number]

Appendix 8: Infertility-Related Diagnosis Codes

792.2	Abnormal Sperm
635.02	Abortion—Complete
637.92	Abortion—Complete
635.01	Abortion—Incomplete
637.91	Abortion—Incomplete
629.9	Abortion—Recurrent
634	Abortion—Spontaneous
640	Abortion—Threatened
646.3	Abortion, Habitual
632	Abortion, Missed
255.3	Adrenal Hyperfunction
255.4	Adrenal Hypofunction
255.2	Adrenogenital Syndrome
626	Amenorrhea
606	Azoospermia
220	Benign Ovarian Tumor/Cyst
622.9	Cervical Disease, Other
616	Cervicitis
V70.0	Complete Exam (Annual)
752.3	Congenital Anomaly
620.1	Cyst—Luteal
620.2	Cyst, Ovarian
620.8	Cyst, Paratubal
595	Cystitis
625.3	Dysmenorrhea
625	Dyspareunia
633.1	Ectopic Pregnancy
621.3	Endometrial Hyperplasia
621	Endometrial Polyp
617.9	Endometriosis
617.8	Endometriosis of Bladder, Vulva
617.2	Endometriosis of Fallopian Tube
617.1	Endometriosis, Ovary
615.9	Endometritis
622	Eversion—Cervix
V723	Exam General/Routine
V72.3	GYN Exam (Annual)
995.2	Hyperstimulation
628.9	Infertility
628.4	Infertility—Cervical
628.2	Infertility—Tubal Origin
628.3	Infertility—with Uterine Factor
628	Infertility Due to Anovulation
626.5	Intermenstrual Bleeding
626.6	Intermenstrual Bleeding

621.5   Intrauterine Adhesions
54.21   Laparoscopy
54.5   Lysis of Adhesions, Peritoneal
606.9   Male Infertility—Unspecified
183   Malignant Neoplasm of Ovary
760.79   Maternal DES/Other
626.1   Menorrhagia
626.2   Menorrhea
626.4   Menses, Irregular
V65.5   Normal
606.1   Oligospermia
752   Ovarian Adhesions
256.8   Ovarian Dysfunction
256.9   Ovarian Dysfunction
256.3   Ovarian Failure
620.5   Ovarian Torsion
614.6   Pelvic Adhesions
614.9   Pelvic Inflammatory Disease

625.9   Pelvic Pain
617.3   Pelvic Peritoneum
627.1   Postmenopausal Bleeding
V72.4   Pregnancy Unconfirmed
V23.0   Pregnancy with History of Infertility
V23.9   Pregnancy, High Risk, Nonspecific
V25.8   Sperm Count Post Vasectomy
614.1   Tubal Obstruction
V26.0   Tuboplasty After Previous Sterilization
608.9   Unspecified Disorder Male Genital Organ
218   Uterine Fibroid—Submucous
619.8   Uterine Fistula
218.9   Uterine Myomata

Appendix 9: Best Places for Infertility Treatments and Family Building

Exceptional fertility clinics and individual fertility specialists can be found throughout the United States. Because of their particular attention to insurance coverage, access to care, and the availability of a wide variety of infertility treatments and family building options, some states are viewed as friendlier when it comes to family building and treating infertility.

We've rated the fifty states plus the District of Columbia as either "Excellent," "Good," "Fair," or "Poor" based on a number of important state-specific criteria, including the number of fertility clinics; ratio of clinics per capita of infertile women; geographic distribution of clinics; number of IVF cycles; number of egg donor cycles; utilization of ICSI, frozen embryos, donor embryos, and gestational carriers; percentage of IVF cycles performed on women over the age of forty; accessibility for single women and gays and lesbians; CDC reporting; highly rated clinics included in the 2005 issue of *Child Magazine*; fertility-friendly companies listed in the 2007 and 2008 issues of *Conceive Magazine*; infertility insurance mandates; family-building laws and regulations; number of adoptions; and the National Council for Adoption's adoption index report. For a full description of our methodology, as well as up-to-date information about fertility care, please visit our website at www.budget ingforinfertility.com.

VERY GOOD	GOOD	FAIR	POOR
Illinois	California	Alabama	Maine
Massachusetts	Connecticut	Alaska	Montana
New Jersey	Delaware	Arizona	Wyoming
New York	District of Columbia	Arkansas	
	Hawaii	Colorado	
	Maryland	Florida	
	Missouri	Georgia	
	New Hampshire	Idaho	
	Ohio	Indiana	
	Oregon	Iowa	
	Rhode Island	Kansas	
	Texas	Kentucky	
	Vermont	Louisiana	
	West Virginia	Michigan	
		Minnesota	
		Mississippi	
		Nebraska	
		Nevada	
		New Mexico	
		North Carolina	
		North Dakota	
		Oklahoma	
		Pennsylvania	
		South Carolina	
		South Dakota	
		Tennessee	
		Utah	
		Virginia	
		Washington	
		Wisconsin	

Appendix 10:
Fertility Bill of Rights

In order to increase the number of excellent places for fertility care and family building, all states should strive for the following:

1. Acknowledge infertility as a disease, lessen the financial burden on families, and improve birth outcomes by supporting insurance coverage for infertility treatments.

2. Ensure all people have access to appropriate fertility care.

3. Respect the diversity of people seeking fertility care, especially with regard to age, gender, diagnosis, race, ethnicity, marital status, and sexual orientation.

4. Promote third-party reproduction as a valuable family building option.

5. Eliminate barriers for families wanting to pursue adoption.

6. Involve infertility patients and solicit their input when considering new guidelines, regulations, or legislation impacting family building options or the treatment of infertility.

Appendix 11: Summary of State Mandates for Insurance Coverage

Since the 1980s, fifteen states—Arkansas, California, Connecticut, Hawaii, Illinois, Louisiana, Maryland, Massachusetts, Montana, New Jersey, New York, Ohio, Rhode Island, Texas, and West Virginia—have passed state laws (also called mandates) requiring insurers to either cover or offer coverage for infertility diagnosis and treatment. Most of these states have laws that require insurance companies to cover infertility treatments at some level (although this level varies dramatically depending on the specific state mandate, employer, and insurance plan). Two states—California and Texas—have laws that require insurance companies only to offer coverage for infertility treatment.

For more information about insurance coverage, please visit our website at www.budgetingforinfertility.com or visit one of these organization's website: American Society for Reproductive Medicine (www.asrm.org) or National Conference of State Legislators (www.ncsl.org).

Arkansas	*Limited Mandate*—This law requires all health insurers that cover maternity benefits to cover the cost of IVF.
California	*Mandate to Offer*—This law requires insurers to offer coverage for infertility and diagnosis, not including IVF.
Connecticut	*Limited Mandate*—This law requires certain insurance plans to provide a one-time only benefit for outpatient costs resulting from IVF.
Hawaii	*Limited Mandate*—This law requires certain insurance plans to provide a one-time only benefit for outpatient costs resulting from IVF.

Illinois	*Comprehensive Mandate*—This law requires insurance policies that cover more than twenty-five people and provide pregnancy-related benefits to cover costs of diagnosis and treatment of infertility.
Louisiana	*Limited Mandate*—The law states that insurers may not deny coverage for treatment of a correctable medical condition to someone solely because the condition results in infertility.
Maryland	*Limited Mandate*—This law requires health and hospital insurance policies that provide pregnancy-related benefits to also cover the outpatient costs of IVF.
Massachusetts	*Comprehensive Mandate*—This law requires health maintenance organizations (HMOs) that cover pregnancy-related benefits to cover medically necessary expenses of infertility diagnosis and treatment.
Montana	*Limited Mandate*—This law requires health maintenance organizations to cover infertility services as part of basic preventative health care services.
New Jersey	*Comprehensive Mandate*—This law requires insurance policies that cover more than fifty people and provide pregnancy-related benefits to cover the cost of diagnosis and treatment of infertility.
New York	*Limited Mandate*—Insurers are required to cover all diagnosis and treatment of correctable medical conditions and shall not exclude coverage of a condition solely because the medical condition results in infertility. This does not include IVF.
Ohio	*Limited Mandate*—This law requires health maintenance organizations (HMOs) to cover basic preventive health services, including infertility.
Rhode Island	*Comprehensive Mandate*—This law requires insurers and health maintenance organizations (HMOs) that cover pregnancy services to cover the cost of medically necessary expenses of diagnosis and treatment of infertility.
Texas	*Mandate to Offer*—This law requires certain insurance that covers pregnancy services to offer coverage for IVF.
West Virginia	*Limited Mandate*—This law requires health maintenance organizations (HMOs) to cover basic health services, including infertility services, when medically necessary.

FAMILY BUILDING FRIENDLY WORKPLACES

Each year the editors at *Conceive Magazine* compile a list of the fifty most fertility-friendly and adoption-friendly workplaces in the United States. To find out if your workplace made this list, visit the *Conceive Magazine* website at www.conceiveonline.com.

Bibliography

Agigian, Amy. 2006. *Baby Steps: How Lesbian Alternative Insemination Is Changing the World.* Middletown, CT: Wesleyan University Press.

Ahuja, K. K., and Simons, E. G. 2006. "Advanced Oocyte Cryopreservation Will Not Undermine the Practice of Ethical Egg Sharing." *Reproductive BioMedicine Online* 12(3): 282–283, www.rbmonline.com/Article/2238 (retrieved 01/19/06).

American Fertility Association. *Trying to Conceive.* www.theafa.org/library/conceive .html (retrieved 12/01/07).

American Society for Reproductive Medicine. *State Infertility Insurance Laws.* www .asrm.org/Patients/insur.html (retrieved 11/15/07).

———. *Frequently Asked Questions About Infertility.* www.asrm.org (retrieved 09/ 21/07).

Appel, Jacob M. 2006. "May Doctors Refuse Infertility Treatments to Gay Patients?" *Hastings Center Report*, September–October.

Barna, Beverly. 2002. *Infertility Sucks! Keeping It All Together When Sperm and Egg Stubbornly Remain Apart.* Xlibris.

The Boston Women's Health Collective. 2005. *Our Bodies, Ourselves.* New York: Touchstone.

Bradford, Stacey. 2007. "How to Cut Your Health-Care Costs." *SmartMoney.* www .smartmoney.com (retrieved 10/06/07).

Brown, Laura Lewis. 2007. "Financing Your Way Through Fertility Treatment." *Revolution Health Group.* www.revolutionhealthgroup.com (retrieved 09/06/07).

Center for Applied Reproductive Science (CARS). *The Learning Center*. www.ivf-et
.com/tlc/archivesintro.html (retrieved 05/10/07).

Centers for Disease Control and Prevention. 2005. *ART Success Rates*. www.cdc.gov/
ART (retrieved 11/15/07).

Chavarro, Jorge E., and Willett, Walter C. 2007. *The Fertility Diet*. New York: McGraw-
Hill.

Collura, Barbara. *Creating a Financial Plan*. www.resolve.org/site/PageServer?pagename
=lrn_mta_finplan (retrieved 11/15/07).

———. *The Costs of Infertility Treatment*. www.resolve.org/site/PageServer?pagename
=lrn?mta?cost&JServSessionIdr007 (retrieved 09/05/07).

Couz, Dr. 2006. *Tales from the Emergency Room and Beyond*. http://drcouz.blogspot
.com/2006/10/allure-of-multiples-i-dont-get-it.html.

Debano, Patty Doyle, Menzel, Courtney Edgerton, and Sutphen, Shelly Dicken. 2005.
The Conception Chronicles. Deerfield Beach, FL: Health Communications, Inc.

Domar, Alice, and Kelly, Alice Lesch. 2004. *Conquering Infertility: Dr. Alice Domar's
Mind/Body Guide to Enhancing Fertility and Coping with Infertility*. New York: Pen-
guin.

Donaldson, Michael C. 2007. *Fearless Negotiating*. New York: McGraw-Hill.

EMD Serono. *Fertility LifeLines: Paying for Your Treatment*. www.fertilitylifelines.com
(retrieved 05/08/07).

———. *Maximizing Your Insurance Coverage for Infertility*. www.fertilitylifelines.com
(retrieved 05/08/07).

Genetics & IVF Institute (GIVF). *Understanding Success Rates*. www.givf.com/success
rates/understandingsuccessrates.cfm (retrieved 12/12/07).

Georgia Reproductive Specialists (GRS). *Your Infertility Home on the Net*. www.ivf.com/
(retrieved 06/03/07).

Glazer, Ellen Sarasohn, and Sterling, Evelina Weidman. 2005. *Having Your Baby
Through Egg Donation*. Indianapolis, IN: Perspectives Press.

Gordon, John D., and DiMattina, Michael. 2007. *100 Questions & Answers About Infertility*. Boston: Jones and Bartlett Publishers.

Griffith, Kelly. July, 2005. "Escape from the Red States: Gay Parents Can Wake Up
to Find That Their Home State Wants to Break Up Their Family. Some Fight Back;
Others Simply Leave for Friendlier Locales." *The Advocate*.

HealthFacts. 1994. *Infertility Treatments: A Demand for More Honesty*. www.encyclo pedia.com (retrieved 1/23/08).

Heng, B. 2007. "Should Fertility Specialists Refer Local Patients Abroad for Shared or Commercialized Oocyte Donation?" *Fertility and Sterility* 87(1): 6–7.

Henne, Melinda, and M. Dale Bundolf. 2008. "Insurance Mandates and Trends in Infertility Treatments." *Fertility and Sterility* 89(1): 66–73.

Holzer, Hananel, Casper, Robert, and Tulandi, Togas. 2006. "A New Era in Ovulation Induction." *Fertility and Sterility* 85(2): 277–284.

Howard, Gary, and Carlson, Dave. 2006. "Financing Options for Assisted Reproductive Technology." *Resolve*. http://www.resolve.org/site/PageServer?pagename=cop _ch_20060208 (retrieved 01/22/08).

The InterNational Council on Infertility Information Dissemination (INCIID). *Complementary Medicine*. www.inciid.org/index.php?page=complementarymed (retrieved 06/15/07).

Jaffe, Jane, David Diamond, and Martha Diamond. 2005. *Unsung Lullabies: Understanding and Coping with Infertility*. New York: St. Martin's Griffin.

Johnson, Patricia Irwin. 2008. *Adopting: Sound Choices, Strong Families*. Indianapolis, IN: Perspectives Press.

Kawada, Yukari. "Reproductive Tourism Trends from Japan." *International Consumer Support for Infertility*. www.icsi.ws (retrieved 11/28/07).

Khamsi, Roxanne. 2007. "Fast Track IVF Saves Time and Lowers Risk." *NewScientist*. www.newscientist.com (retrieved 11/28/07).

Mackon, Nick S., et al. "The Science Behind 25 Years of Ovarian Stimulation for in Vitro Fertilization." *Endocrine Reviews* 27(2): 170–207.

March of Dimes. 2006. *Estimated Costs of Prematurity in the United States*. http://www .marchofdimes.com/prematurity/21198_15349asp.

Margolis, Cindy. 2008. *Having a Baby . . . When the Old-Fashioned Way Isn't Working*. New York: A Perigee Book.

Martin, Justin. 2003. "A Baby or Your Money Back Is Dr. Geoffrey Sher's Fertility Clinic's Promise Results and Deliver Profits. Some Rivals Find His Methods Unseemly. Others Imitate Them." *CNN Money Online*. www.cnnmoney.com (retrieved 11/27/07).

Mayes, Gwen. 2003. "Infertility Insurance Laws." *Infertility Times*, 1.

Medical News Today. 2007. "Pregnancy Without Multiple Births Enabled by New

IVF Technique." *Medical News Today Online*. www.medicalnewstoday.com (retrieved 10/02/07).

Mundy, Liza. 2007. *Everything Conceivable: How the Science of Assisted Reproduction Is Changing Our World*. New York: Knopf.

Nadeau, Jenna Currier. 2007. *The Empty Picture Frame: An Inconceivable Journey Through Infertility*. Outskirts Press. www.inconceivablejourney.com.

National Institutes of Health. *Understanding Clinical Trials*. www.asrm.org/Patients/insur.html (retrieved 11/15/08).

Orin, Rhonda. 2001. *Make Them Pay: How to Get the Most from Health Insurance and Managed Care*. New York: St. Martin's Griffin.

Panayotov, Jodi. *In Vitro Fertility Goddess*. www.invitrofertilitygoddess.com.

Parker-Pope, Tara. 2007. "Can a 'Fertility Diet' Get You Pregnant?" *The New York Times*, December 18.

Pascual, Psyche. 2002. "Financing Infertility Treatments." *Caremark*. http://health resources.caremark.com/topic/infertilityfinance (retrieved 01/22/08).

Paulson, Richard J., and Sachs, Judith. 1998. *Rewinding Your Biological Clock: Motherhood Late in Life*. New York: W. H. Freeman and Company.

RESOLVE. *Evaluating Infertility Treatment Financing Plans*. www.resolve.org (retrieved 8/05/07).

———. *Insurance Coverage Facts*. www.resolve.org/site/PageServer?pagename=ta_ic_icf (retrieved 11/15/07).

Richards, Sarah E. 2007. "Skipping Baby Steps: The Case for Going Straight to IVF." *Slate*. www.slate.com (retrieved 11/21/07).

Roberts, MacKenna. 2008. "IVF Clinics Should Give Personalized Costed Treatment Plans." *The [London] Times*. http://business.timesonline.co.uk (retrieved 1/14/08).

Roizen, Michael F., and Oz, Mehmet C. 2006. *You the Smart Patient—An Insider's Handbook for Getting the Best Treatment*. New York: Free Press.

Schlosberg, Suzanne. 2007. *The Essential Fertility Log*. Cambridge, MA: DaCapo.

Schmittlein, David C., and Morrison, Donald G. 1999. *A Live Baby or Your Money Back: The Marketing of In Vitro Fertilization Procedures*. Unpublished.

Sember, Brette McWhorter. 2004. *The Complete Adoption and Fertility Legal Guide*. Naperville, IL: Sphinx Publisher.

Sloan, Louise. 2007. *Knock Yourself Up: A Tell-All Guide to Becoming a Single Mother.* New York: Avery.

Society for Assisted Reproduction. *IVF Success Rates Reports.* www.sart.org/ (retrieved 08/03/07).

Spar, Debora. 2006. *The Baby Business: How Money, Science and Politics Drive the Commerce of Conception.* Boston: Harvard Business School Press.

Swire-Falker, Elizabeth. 2004. *Infertility Survival Handbook.* New York: Riverhead Trade.

Thatcher, Samuel. *ART Success Rates: All That Glimmers.* www.ivf-et.com/tlc/fact_art _success.html (retrieved 12/10/07).

Vargo, Julie, and Regan, Maureen. 2005. *A Few Good Eggs: Two Chicks Dish on Overcoming the Insanity of Infertility.* New York: ReganBooks.

Weschler, Toni. 2002. *Taking Charge of Your Fertility: The Definitive Guide to Natural Birth Control, Pregnancy Achievement and Reproductive Health.* New York: Quill.

Woodman, Josef. 2007. *Patients Beyond Borders: Everybody's Guide to Affordable, World-Class Medical Tourism.* Chapel Hill, NC: Healthy Travel Media.

Index

EVELINA WEIDMAN STERLING is an accomplished and well-known infertility expert, public health educator, and researcher. She is currently the CEO of My Fertility Plan (www.myfertilityplan.com), a leading infertility consulting firm aimed at providing health care consumers and infertility patients with a wide range of unbiased and evidence-based educational resources and referrals. My Fertility Plan helps patients better navigate through their fertility care and encourages informed decision-making.

Evelina has co-written several other bestselling and award-winning books focusing on reproductive health, including *Living with Polycystic Ovary Syndrome* (Addicus Books, 2000), *Having Your Baby through Egg Donation* (Perspectives Press, 2005), and *Before Your Time: Living Well with Early Menopause* (Simon & Schuster, 2010). Evelina has also published several articles and has given numerous interviews and presentations about various aspects of fertility, including the many complex issues associated with overcoming infertility.

Evelina holds a Ph.D. in Medical Sociology from Georgia State University as well as a master's degree in Public Health from the Johns Hopkins University. She also attended the University of Mary Washington where she earned a Bachelor of Science degree in Biology. Evelina has over fifteen years of experience working in public health education and research, primarily in the areas of reproductive and women's health. Previous experience includes positions at Healthy Mothers, Healthy Babies National Coalition, American Association for Health Education, Health Resources and Services Administration, Gallaudet University, and the American Heart Association. She also regularly serves as an independent consultant helping nonprofit organizations and government agencies effectively develop, implement, and evaluate public health and health education programs.

Evelina is passionate and committed to providing all families with the tools they need to grow their families. She lives in Atlanta with her husband and two children (who were conceived with the assistance of fertility treatments).

ANGIE BEST-BOSS is an award-winning women's health writer and is a passionate infertility consumer advocate. In addition to co-authoring *Living with Polycystic Ovary Syndrome* (Addicus Books, 2000), Angie has written three other books, including *The Everything Digestive Health Book*. She has a Bachelor's of Arts degree in Sociology and Journalism from Virginia Wesleyan College and a Masters of Divinity degree with an emphasis in counseling from Union Theological Seminary.

Her articles on women's health and infertility have appeared in dozens of both online and print resources, including *MD News, Massage Therapy Today, Family Building Magazine,* conceivingconcepts.com, obgyn.net, iparenting.com, pcosupport.org. She is lead medical writer for www.conceivingconcepts.com and is a member of the American Medical Writers Association. She is a featured blogger at How to Make a Family: Baby-Making from Every Conceivable Angle (http://howtomakeafamily.typepad.com/).

Angie lives in New Palestine, Indiana, with her husband and three daughters. After being diagnosed with PCOS, Angie used a variety of medical and alternative treatments to conceive.

To contact Evelina or Angie, you may visit their website at
www.myfertilityplan.com
or call them toll-free at 877–509-PLAN.